Holy Crap I Have Cancer!
Now What?

What to Expect When You Weren't Expecting

Ann Low

Dedicated to:
YOU! ♥

Disclaimer

Hey there, you daring reader!

So, here's the deal with this book—it's all about cancer, and it's packed with the thoughts and ideas of yours truly. Now, don't get me wrong, I'm not a medical guru or anything close to that. I'm just a regular person with a penchant for sarcasm, cheekiness, and irreverence, trying to dish out some informative stuff

Listen up! This book is NOT a substitute for professional medical advice, health expertise, or any personal services. So, before you go all-in on any of the suggestions I've sprinkled in these pages or start drawing conclusions, make sure you consult a real-deal medical or health expert. I mean, seriously, it's your health we're talking about here—better be safe than sorry!

Now, pay attention—I'm washing my hands of any responsibility for whatever you do with the information in this book. Whether it's a liability, loss, or some bizarre risk that pops up as a result of your actions, it's on you, my friend. I mean, we're just having some sarcastic fun here, but life is serious business, so take it seriously, okay?

There you have it. Use your common sense, be smart, and keep that health in check. Stay sassy and informed, but always seek the advice of the pros when it comes to the serious stuff. And remember, I'm just a quirky survivor trying to help you out, not a certified doctor or anything!

Love and laughter,
Ann Low

CONTENTS

INTRODUCTION

You've just heard the "C" word. NO! Not the dirty one!

The one that is even worse. . .

CANCER.

If you are reading this book, I suspect that either you (or someone you care deeply about) has just become a member in a club that you never asked to join, with dues that can be physically, mentally, and financially staggering.

You've been diagnosed with cancer.

Cancer is like having children: There is no owner's manual. No playbook. There is no one who prepares us for how to "do" cancer.

Don't get me wrong — there are plenty of great books out there and tons of literature available. The problem is that often the books, although great and informative, are long, and during the flurry of activity a cancer diagnosis brings in the beginning, you often don't have time to read them until you are already deeply into treatment. By that time, the questions you may have had at diagnosis, you have already figured out, forgot to ask or you were forced to learn the hard way . . . by experience.

The other challenge I had with some of the piles of literature I received is that everyone looked so happy and upbeat. In the photos were the attractive smiling doctors wearing their lab coats, with their stethoscopes hanging loosely around their necks. Standing with them is the smiling couple, who looked like they are about to get into the Cialis bathtub, rather than looking like they just received news that will turn their world, as they know it, upside down.

Quite frankly, those upbeat doctors and smiling faces were not the reality for me, nor for most cancer patients and survivors whom I have spoken with. I was so surprised and shocked that I recall very few smiles. I felt more like the Edvard Munch painting of *The Scream* than these smiling rays of sunshine in the literature that I was handed by the armful. I hated seeing those happy faces when it didn't occur for me as a smile-worthy experience.

It was scary.

It was confusing.

It was me spending about 30 days outside of my body, kind of watching everything happening as if it was happening to someone else.

I felt like one of those toys you wind up that just walks around and bumps into walls and turns around and does it again and again and again.

It was a very strange experience, and as I have talked to hundreds of other patients and survivors, they share many of the same feelings. Perhaps worded differently, but still that out-of-body, what-in–the-world-is-happening-to-me experience.

I have always said about myself that I'm spontaneous as long as I have a couple of weeks to plan for it. I wanted to know ahead of time what to expect and how to prepare for this new thing called Ann's Cancer. I didn't want to be the person that was frequently saying things to myself like..." I wish I had known that before I_____" (insert anything like: before I had surgery, chemotherapy, lopped off a body part or two.) or "I wish someone had told me_____" (insert anything like: I didn't have to rush my decision, I had time.)

Fortunately, I didn't have to say that to myself too often. Just a few days after I was diagnosed, an acquaintance of mine insisted we meet for coffee. Terry and I had been acquainted for several years through a mutual friend, had spent a Thanksgiving meal together, were friends on Facebook, and had been trying to meet for coffee for a couple of those years. Apparently, we weren't trying very hard because it took my cancer diagnosis to finally make it occur.

Terry was one of those individuals that when she texts you to meet her, you do, as she always has so much to offer. This was a female attorney who sat on the sub-committees investigating the assassinations of both John F. Kennedy and Martin Luther King, Jr. Later she was instrumental in beginning sponsorships with sports teams — primarily the NFL — something that today is a multi-billion-dollar industry.

Oh...and she was in Year 5 of a terminal cancer diagnosis, where she had originally been given just six months to live.

This was someone that had the resources to seek the best medical care and treatments in the world. Someone who was willing to sit and share with me what to expect, the do's, and the don't-bothers. Plus, she was willing to answer any questions I might have, regardless of how stupid.

I leapt at the opportunity to meet with her and spent several hours picking her brain and asking an array of questions while taking extensive notes.

Our family calls ourselves the Lucky Lows, and I feel incredibly lucky for having connected with Terry. Without a doubt I felt those hours I spent with Terry made my own cancer journey so much easier by having me be somewhat prepared for what to expect. I felt I was so lucky to have had that opportunity to be coached and mentored by someone who had walked the journey before me. And not just walked the journey, but had walked over burning coals to be where she was.

All through my treatment, I wished **everyone** had access to a Terry, as I met so many people who faced many surprises because they clearly either didn't understand things, hadn't been told, or hadn't asked. Things I already knew, so they were not a surprise to me because Terry had prepared me, and I was a little more knowledgeable about the process because of her sharing of information.

Once I completed active treatment, and met others that were new to the journey, it became even more obvious that everyone could use a coach or an owner's manual.

That's when I realized that there **was** that possibility. That everyone **could** have the knowledge.

I realized that I could share Terry's wisdom and my own experiences in a short book, so that perhaps others could be empowered for their journey. Something short. Something to prepare a patient at least a little for what they might face and experience over the next 30, 60, or 90 days. The days when a patient is first trying to get the hang of this thing called CANCER.

That is what you hold in your hands now — a guide of what to expect when you weren't expecting to hear, "I'm sorry but you have cancer."

I wanted to create something that, if you were diagnosed with cancer today, you could purchase or download and quickly read it and have a better idea of what might be ahead for you. Things that might help you feel a little **more in control** during a time when you often feel like you have little control.

Even with a background in the medical industry, prior to my diagnosis, what I knew about cancer would fit on the head of a pin and have plenty of room left over. I'm sure, even now, that I don't fully understand much of it, as it can be quite complicated. But I do know enough to hopefully guide you through the things that are going to occur over the next few weeks, or months, and to offer some advice that I learned from others, or that helped me personally. There are going to be specific tests and other things that I share here that may not apply to your particular cancer. But for many of you, it will give you some idea of things that could possibly be ahead for you, how to prepare for them, and what to expect.

If knowledge is power, then sharing your knowledge empowers others and that's what I hope this book does for you - empowers you on this journey. If it helps just one person's journey be a little bit easier, than I will feel like I have written the greatest bestseller ever!

• • •

The best way to use this book is to **read each short chapter FIRST**. At the end of each chapter are some *Tips* and then my story. I would **definitely** read the *Tips*, as they are things that will help along the way. I've also included some *Ann's Tips.* These are remedies I learned along the way on my own, from other survivors, others in treatment, oncology doctors and nurses. Those I tried that personally helped me and many others, I have included in *Ann's Tips* as I felt they were worth sharing.

*This is where the medical disclaimer comes in. **ALWAYS** run any of these suggestions by your medical professional first. I am not a doctor and any suggestions you glean from this book (or any of your helpful friends who will inundate you with information about how to eat, where to get coffee enemas, what new therapies you must try and all the internet cures) **should be run by your physician first.** If you don't like any of these suggestions, DO NOT DO THEM. I learned quickly not to base **MY** decisions on the advice of those who didn't have to deal with the results, or hadn't been there and done that.

After getting through the chapters and the tips, you can either read my story or skip over it, as it isn't pertinent to the purpose of the book. Empowering you with what might be ahead for you over the next few months is really the most important thing so read the Chapters and Tips first. My story is just there to share my journey. (**As we are all unique, so is our journey. Mine was not particularly easy as I have other underlying health conditions – both autoimmune issues and a history of infections - that made mine a bit more challenging. *Yours will be completely different!)* **What is the most important is to review the information that might have you better prepared for what you are about to face, regardless of whether you are a Stage 0 or a Stage IV.**

I do have to issue a PG-13 ***warning***. This book is written with some foul language and maybe even some distasteful humor, so it's quite possible that this might not be for everyone. (I had to find humor in all of this or I'm pretty sure I wouldn't have gotten through it.) If you are easily offended by words like ass, shit, fuck, or damn, then this book may not be for you. But I learned very early on with a cancer diagnosis that foul language has its place . . . it's maybe even necessary for some of us, as this trip is truly a life-altering journey worthy of a few cuss words here and there. And know that for most of us, if we aren't saying it out loud, we are certainly uttering it in our heads.

If you can get past that, my hope is this book has enough information that it eases your journey a bit, perhaps makes you smile, and helps you realize there are others just like you. . . people who have fought the good fight and are willing to assist you in being as prepared as you can possibly be, so you are empowered to fight the good fight as well.

Now sit down, suit up, and prepare for the game!

Your Cancer Coach,
~ Ann ♥

My Story: B.C. (Before Cancer)

I'm not a doctor and I don't play one on TV.

And I'm not famous. Not a movie star, sports figure, or anyone well known.

I'm probably just like you - unless, of course, you are a doctor, you play one on TV, or you're famous. Then I'm not just like you.

But chances are you and I probably have a lot in common.

I'm just an everyday person.

I'm a daughter, a sister, and a wife. I've grown two humans in my uterus and pushed them out of my vagina; and despite me, they have turned out to be incredibly amazing people.

I had an over 20-year career in the health care in clinical medicine. I'm incredibly grateful for that experience as it gave me enough knowledge to often make me a real pain in the ass to my doctors and insurance companies. That knowledge has enabled me to ask questions that others might not even think to ask.

In 1996, I left my career to stay home to have my kids raise me. And raise me well, they did.

I was a room mom and a high school lacrosse coach. I've been on field trips, attended school band concerts, and never missed a school function. I answered phones at the high school and lost count of the number of sporting events I've attended.

I'm a partner in a Commercial General Contracting Construction business that has been successful since 2007, where I sleep with the boss, my husband. 2007 was not a great time to start a construction business in Arizona, but here we are more than a decade later, still around.

And like many folks, I had gained and lost the same 60 pounds for the past 25 years. I am a human accordion. . .lose, gain, lose, gain, lose, gain more.

I have also helped run Little League Baseball here in our area for more than 15 years. (You'll see that throughout this book I equate some of this journey to the terms, analogies, and idioms from Little League and baseball. This frame of reference worked for me as Little League has been such an important part of my life and I was at the end of one season and beginning another when I was diagnosed. It helped me be a little entertained in trying to make some sense of this often-crazy journey.)

Mostly, I've been busy living my life with the goal to get my kids through debtor's prison — college — and to eventually ride off into the sunset with my wonderful husband, Hubby.

2011 was a pivotal year for me. That's the year I turned 50. Yup — the big Five-Oh. Turning fifty didn't bother me in the slightest. My father and sister were both deceased prior to their 40th birthdays, so I figured each year I lived past 40 put me WAY ahead in the game.

However, I wasn't blind to the fact that I really needed to take a very serious look at my health if, indeed, I wanted to ride off into that sunset with that Hubby.

And not just a look. I needed to seriously do something about it. I was easily 40, but probably more like 50, pounds overweight. For long periods, I would eat like a yoga instructor and would lose a few pounds, to only return to eating like a crazed kid in a candy store and gain it all, and more, back. I was on high blood pressure and high cholesterol medications. My knees ached and I had suffered my entire adult life with migraines. Plus, I come from a long line of relatives that have died from cardiac episodes. I knew I was heading down that exact same path if I didn't make some significant changes. Actually, my exam with my cardiologist that year indicated that I wasn't just heading toward that path. . .I had already rounded first base and was well on my way to second.

My exercise routine seemed to follow the same cycle. I would exercise like a fiend before getting injured and needing to take a break from exercise to heal, only to repeat the same pattern a few weeks or months down the road.

But basically, I pretty much felt like shit. Tired all the time and craving foods that weren't good for me. I was caught in the cycle of being depressed about my weight, but not keeping it off; feeling depressed because I couldn't keep it off; reverting to eating everything in sight because I was depressed, causing me to add more weight, which just added to the depression.

Perhaps you can relate. If not, I'm jealous as hell.

The year I turned 50, with both of our kids safely enrolled in college, I no longer had my kids to use as an excuse for not taking better care of myself. I decided to take a year and make some significant, and what would hopefully be, life-long health changes. No quick fixes. No fad diets. No pills or potions. Just good old-fashioned resolve to eat better and exercise more — and do both more intelligently.

I started following a modified Paleo diet and hired a personal trainer. I became a permanent fixture at the gym at 9:00 a.m. on Monday, Wednesday, and Friday and I hiked or walked the other days, while resting on Sundays. I followed the advice of putting my exercise on the calendar and I lived by it. Other than the most important of things, that exercise routine became MY time and everyone who relied on me knew it and supported it.

And it paid off. Big time!

In June of 2014 I reached my goal weight, was in the best physical shape of my life, and under my doctor's guidance, I was able to discontinue all my medications. I was making plans for running a half-marathon and was looking at the obstacle course races that I wanted to enter over the next year. I felt badass! Fit and ready to take on the world. I even had people asking me how I had done it, so I'd started doing what I love to do, which is to coach and support others in reaching THEIR goals to be better.

But I also had a little nagging issue. Nothing serious — but annoying. I had begun doing more of a CrossFit workout, which meant there were some really intense workouts where I might be more sore than other times. REALLY sore. That soreness would always go away as I recovered; with the exception of one area that never seemed to stop bothering me. It wasn't real pain — I was just constantly aware that the lymph nodes under my left arm constantly bothered me. Sometimes they seemed swollen, but most of the time they were just sore to the touch. Since I had made my health a priority, I decided it was time to have it checked out when it didn't resolve.

There I was, up to bat, waiting for a nice, fat, over-the-plate pitch, so I could swing for the fences. Instead, I received an unexpected curveball, where my life took a surprising turn and my journey through cancer began.

INSURANCE (Rookie Eligibility)

Per Major Leagues Baseball's collective bargaining agreement, players must meet certain criteria in order to be eligible for play.

The same thing can be said for you with your insurance. You need to know your eligibility and fully understand the details of your insurance plan before you put your cancer team together, as your insurance may dictate who you can see and where you can be treated.

From your first doctor visit, where you are suspicious something might be wrong, all the way through to Survivorship, the cruise we all want to go on, insurance will be the ONLY constant. *Every step of the way!*

In order to make sure you get the best possible treatment, you've got to fully understand what services are covered on YOUR insurance, or what procedures you must follow in order to get the therapy you require.

What are the rules? What kind of pitches might you be looking at? How do I get on base? What happens if I strike out?

Because, quite honestly, the costs of **NOT** understanding your health insurance coverage can be financially devastating.

So, don your jock strap and put on your cleats for a short lesson in this thing we call Health Insurance. (This relates only to insurance in the United States and some of this information may have changed depending on when you are reading this. If you are in another country, you will need to educate yourself to its nuances, so you get the best treatment and coverage available to you.)

Health Insurance

Health insurance coverage pays for provider services, diagnostic testing, blood work, hospital care, and medications. How much of that care and how many of those services it will pay for depends on the type of coverage you have. That is why it is imperative that you know your insurance coverage before you have *any* treatment or therapies, as cancer treatment, regardless of the type of cancer, can be quite expensive.

There are different types of health insurance plans and coverage. The most common plan types include HMOs (Health Maintenance Organizations), PPOs (Preferred Provider Organizations) and Medicare.

The things you need to be most familiar with are your:

- Premium
- Co-pay
- Deductible
- Co-insurance
- Out-of-Pocket Maximum
- In Network
- Out-of-Network
- PPO
- HMO
- Covered Services
- Exclusions
- Drug Formulary
- Explanation of Benefits

Premium

This is the amount you pay your insurance company for the privilege of having insurance. You may have the option of paying your premium annually, quarterly, or monthly. Health insurance premiums vary greatly depending on what medical expenses the plan covers, which doctors you can see, and how much you must pay when you use medical services. In general, if you pay a **higher** premium upfront, you will pay **less** when you receive medical care, and vice versa; the **lower** the premium, the **more** you must pay for medical treatment out of your own pocket.

Co-pay

This is one of the ways you share in your medical costs. This is usually a fixed dollar amount you pay for routine services and certain types of care defined by your health plan. For example, your plan might have a co-pay of $20 for a regular doctor visit and a co-pay of $40 to see a Specialist. You may also be charged a co-pay for visiting an emergency room or for purchasing prescription medications. Plans with **higher** premiums generally have **lower** co-pays.

Deductible

This is the annual amount you must **first** pay, out-of-pocket, before coverage kicks in and the insurance company starts paying their contracted portion of your medical bills. For example: If your deductible is $2000, then you would be required to pay the first $2000 in health care treatment that you receive, *each year*, before the insurance company would start paying *any portion of covered services*. Deductibles are determined by the insurance company and are usually set at rounded amounts such as $2000, $4000, or $5500. Typically, the **higher** the premium, the **lower** the deductible. If you decide to seek care for services NOT COVERED by your insurance plan, **these medical bills would NOT be applied to the deductible or the Out-of-Pocket Maximum.**

Co-insurance

This term refers to the portion of your medical bills that you will be responsible for paying when you receive any medical treatment, once your annual deductible has been met. Co-insurance is a type of cost sharing in which you pay a percentage of the cost of your health care and your health insurance company pays for the rest, as long as the services are covered under your plan. Co-insurance kicks in *after* you have met your annual deductible. (This does not include your monthly premium.) Co-insurance is usually a pre-determined percentage of the total covered bill. You often hear it referred to as an 80/20, a 70/30 or even a 50/50 plan.

Let's say you have a plan that has a $2000 deductible and is an 80/20 plan. That means that once you have paid the entire $2000 of your annual deductible, from that point forward, your insurance will pay 80 percent of the ensuing bills and you will be responsible for only 20 percent of those bills until you have reached your Out-of-Pocket Maximum, as long as you are seeing doctors contracted with your insurance company.

Out-of-Pocket Maximum

This is an important part of your insurance, as it is the largest amount of money you pay toward the cost of your health care each year. After you've paid your set amounts in deductibles, co-pays, and co-insurance to reach your out-of-pocket maximum, your health insurance company then pays for the rest of your health care covered services for that year.

But this is where you need to fully understand your insurance as your policy may or may not credit deductibles, co-payments, and co-insurance for some tests to reach your out-of-pocket maximum. Let's stick with the previous example of a plan that has a $2000 deductible and is an 80/20 plan and, let's say, it has a $5000 out-of-pocket maximum. If you have a policy that **includes** deductibles and co-pays you would pay $2000 out-of-pocket toward the deductible and then 20 percent of all your covered services until you reach $5000 in order to meet your out-of-pocket maximum. So, a total out-of-pocket cost to you of $5000. However, if you have an insurance plan that **excludes** deductibles toward your out-of-pocket maximum, you would need to pay a total of $7000 before your insurance company would start paying for all your covered medical expenses.

It's important to fully understand your policy's out-of-pocket terms. If you have any questions about it, call your insurance company for clarification.

In Network

This is the term that refers to doctors, pharmacies, hospitals, and medical establishments who are *contracted* to cover services under your insurance plan. These entities have agreed to the terms of your insurance company and have contracted amounts they have agreed to accept for medical treatment.

Out-of-Network

These are doctors, pharmacies, hospitals, and medical establishments who *do not* participate in your health insurance and are **NOT** contracted by your health insurance company. For services from these entities, you will be responsible for paying for *everything* out of your own pocket.

HMO — Health Maintenance Organization

An HMO type of insurance plan is a medical plan which offers health care services only with specific HMO providers. Under most HMO plans you must first choose a primary care physician and *that* physician will refer you to the other HMO specialists you will require that are within your plan. HMOs require the use of specific, in-network plan providers. Services from providers outside of your HMO plan are rarely ever covered. If you choose to go outside of your HMO plan ALL your care would be your financial responsibility.

PPO — Preferred Provider Organization

In a PPO, the plan contracts with doctors and hospitals to provide services. You must see doctors and get services from providers that are contracted with your insurance company for those costs to be covered. But you usually do not have to see your primary care physician first to arrange all your appointments, as required in an HMO. Like an HMO, if you choose to go outside of your PPO plan ALL your care would be your financial responsibility.

Covered Services

This refers to services or supplies that your health insurance will "cover" (or pay for). They may pay for all or a portion of the cost depending on the terms of your insurance. Most health insurances do not cover all services and supplies, so it is important to educate yourself about any limitations and restrictions that might apply to your plan.

Exclusions

These are often specific services or circumstances in which your insurance plan will not provide **any** benefits. These are exclusions and you will want to familiarize yourself with them.

Drug Formulary

This is a list of prescription medications that are covered by your insurance plan and at what percentage they will pay for specific medications. A formulary varies greatly depending on your insurance provider and the plan you have chosen. Many prescription plans have a deductible you must meet first before they will begin paying for your medications. Medications NOT on your insurance plan formulary will be entirely your responsibility. (If you've been prescribed a drug that is NOT on your formulary and is too expensive for you to manage, reach back out to the prescribing physician to see if there is a substitute that IS covered by your insurance. Although it is time consuming, this could save you thousands of dollars!)

Explanation of Benefits

This is the health insurance company's written explanation of how a medical claim was processed and paid. It contains detailed information about what the company reimbursed your physician, facility, or pharmacy, if there are any contracted adjustments and what portion of the costs you are responsible for.

• • •

Unless you are blessed with abundant resources that makes having insurance just an added benefit, for most of you, your insurance will determine who your team of providers may be, where you can be treated, and how much money you will need to pay and to whom. Your health benefits can vary greatly depending on the type of coverage you have. It is imperative that you **FULLY** understand *YOUR* insurance, preferably before you seek any treatment, so you aren't saddled with undue expenses from the beginning. Knowing everything about your insurance, and being organized from the very beginning, will lessen the stress of the paperwork, which quite frankly can sometimes be incredibly overwhelming. Your insurance will become an important, and often very time-consuming, constant part of this journey.

• • •

Tips:

This journey — regardless of the stage of your cancer — will generate an incredible amount of paperwork. Starting this journey with being organized will assist you as you begin to receive EOBs (Explanation of Benefits), reports, lab results and bills. Being organized will ease things as you go to your different doctor appointments where you will be repeatedly asked many of the same questions. It is very helpful to have everything right at your fingertips, whether at your doctor visits or on the telephone with the insurance company.

I found the best way to stay organized was to create **TWO** 3-ring binders to hold all this information; one for your health records and one for your insurance and billing information.

BINDER 1:

I utilized the first binder for all my personal health information, reports, and lab work. I named it _BOOBS_ but label it any way you like to differentiate it from your second binder that will hold all of your insurance information. _**Take this binder to all your doctor appointments.**_ I assure you that having all this information in one convenient place will be very advantageous. This is also incredibly useful should you have a medical emergency. Someone can just grab this binder and even if you are in no condition to answer questions, and the person taking you to the ER has **no** idea of your situation and history, ALL the important, pertinent information a hospital or doctor would need is readily available.

Suggested Tabs

- **Medical History:** Complete and keep a copy of a medical history form in your binder. (For a copy of one, download from www.holycrapihavecancer.com and complete the Personal and Medical Information Form.) Use it as a reference whenever you go to a doctor and you are asked to complete forms. Keep it up to date with any changes in your history or medication as you move forward.

- **Medications:** Keep an up-to-date list of these on a separate page as they may be changed frequently during treatment. Keep a list of all medications, dosages, and frequency. If a medication is changed or discontinued, do not eliminate it from the list. Cross it off and make a note of when it was changed or discontinued, and why. This is useful if you are sent to a specialist and they ask if you have ever used a specific medication. You can refer to this list and respond accordingly.

- **Advanced Directives:** If you do not have one yet, complete any advance directive forms (living will, medical power of attorney, Do Not Resuscitate) and make a copy to keep in this binder. You will be asked if you have these at pretty much every doctor appointment or hospital visit. Keep a copy in this binder, but do not give it away. If you do not have one, they are usually available from doctors, hospitals, lawyers, libraries, on line, your local Area Agency on Aging or your state health department.

- **Insurance Cards:** It seems that regardless of how often you see the doctor, they will ask to see your insurance card/s nearly every time you are there. Keep copies in this binder in case of an emergency, but also make sure you carry the original as most offices now take advantage of technology and will scan your cards when you come into the office.

- *Calendar* — The longer that active treatment occurs, the harder it is to keep things straight. Keeping an up-to-date calendar, with space to write, is incredibly beneficial. There are plenty of calendars that are available online to download. Be sure to make extra copies of the blank calendar pages for future use. With space to write, a calendar can be used to keep track of eating habits, sleeping patterns, and exercise routines. It can also be used for medication reminders. Although if you have a smartphone there are apps that can assist even better with medication reminders.

- **Notes/Log/Diary:** Keep a running log of your appointments and a diary of your care. You might need it to refer to should you be required to share information regarding when a procedure took place, when a specific test was done, or when a medication was changed.

- **Radiation:** Keep a separate log of the treatment and side effects (if any) if radiation becomes part of your treatment plan. It's easier to refer directly to that section should you want to share information with your doctor, rather than trying to find it in your notes.

- **Chemotherapy:** Keep a separate log of the treatment and side effects (if any) if chemotherapy becomes part of your treatment plan. Chemotherapy tends to follow the same pattern and as the treatment goes on it's easier to forget the experience of the previous cycle. With notes, you will be able to remember what to expect with each cycle of treatment. Also, your oncologist may want you to record specific information such as temperature or rating of any side effects. It's easier to refer directly to that section, should you need to share information with your doctor, rather than trying to find it in your notes.

- **Questions:** This is a great place to keep the list of questions you will want to ask your doctors as you see them. (Go to www.holycrapihavecancer.com for a copy of suggested questions to ask your surgeon, radiation oncologist, or medical oncologist. These are especially useful for your initial visits.)

- **Reports and Scans** — Copies of any of your tests, scans, or reports are important to have in your possession. We are lucky to live in an era where we have so much technology at our fingertips; however, sometimes that technology does not ALWAYS work in our favor. You will want to make sure you have copies of every test result, scan, or bloodwork report you can get your hands on that pertains to your diagnosis and treatment.

  - **Always** ask for copies of your tests, scans, and reports. Sometimes they can be given to you at the time of the appointment; but more often it can take several days to have access to the results. Keep in contact with where you had the test performed, until you receive a copy of the results for your records. (**It can be helpful to ask for the name and direct telephone number of the contact person in that department,**

so you have someone to talk to directly.) Some tests results are only available on a CD. If that is the case, ask for a copy of the CD or see if they will put it on a flash drive that you offer to provide. **(My experience was that sometimes the doctor I was scheduled to see had not received the results of a test or scan, and had I not had a copy with me at the time, the visit would have had to be rescheduled.)** Make sure you are prepared for your visit by having your own copies of the tests performed. You will learn that you must be proactive enough in your care to be prepared for your next appointment. There is SO MUCH waiting that occurs with a cancer diagnosis, that any additional waiting you can avoid reduces stress and frustration. Three-hole punch these reports and add them to your binder. If it is a CD, find a plastic sleeve to file it in. **The best way to file them is by date of service with the most recent in the front.**

- **Labs:** Always ask for copies of your laboratory and blood work results. As more doctors' offices embrace technology, they are creating patient portals where you can often access your lab work online. Some lab work is done right in the doctor's office and you can even get a copy before you leave. If that is the case, make sure you ask for a copy. If it isn't available at the time, stay in contact with the lab until you receive a copy. Again, ask for the name of the contact person so you can stay in touch with the responsible person. Three-hole punch these and add them to your binder. **The best way to file them is by date of service with the most recent in the front.**

DO NOT EVER GIVE YOUR BINDER CONTENTS AWAY! If any of your physicians or nurses need a copy of any part of your binder, have them make a copy and return the original document to you.

BINDER 2:

Utilize the second binder exclusively for your insurance information. I named mine *Insurance* (pretty creative, huh?). Regardless of the extent of your cancer, it will generate an incredible amount of insurance paperwork. This binder is for **that** paperwork only. Do not take it to your appointments unless you are having a specific financial issue with a particular office and you need the information to refer to in order to clear things up.

Suggested Tabs:

- **Policy:** Keep a copy of your insurance policy to refer to if needed. Most insurance companies have an overview *that can be printed.*

- ***Copy of Insurance Cards:*** Keep copies of your insurance card/s in here. Sometimes you are on the phone with someone and you might need to refer to information located on the front or back of your insurance card. It's also useful to have a copy, as that often speeds up the paperwork process, when seeing a new doctor, if you can fax or email them a copy of the front and back of your insurance card.

- **EOBs:** Explanation of Benefits will come to you from your insurance company for every visit, procedure, and medication that is run through your insurance plan. Consider that just one diagnostic test can generate a separate EOB from the facility, physician, anesthesiologist (if one is required), pathologist, and the pharmacy, if you need any medications during or after the test. So, yes that can mean possibly five different documents for just one visit. You can see, by this example, how paperwork can rapidly accumulate. The best way to file EOBs is by date of service, with the most recent in the front. I also recommend that you highlight the date of service, the provider's name, and the amount you owe. This will be helpful when you match them with the bills you will receive, or you need them to refer to for some other reason.

- **Bills:** Keep bills separated until you receive the Explanation of Benefits that coincides with that particular bill. If you receive a bill and have not received the EOB, contact your insurance company as EOBs often arrive before you receive a bill from your doctor. (Again, technology has made many advances and often you can go to your insurance carrier's website and download the EOB.) Then match the EOB with the coinciding bill. Be sure to compare the charges. You do not want to pay a bill without first associating the two to make sure no mistakes have been made. If there is a mistake in the billing, contact the provider and ask them to make the correction and resubmit the bill correctly to your insurance company. If there is a mistake on the EOB, contact your insurance company, explain the mistake, and ask them to correct it. This also may require contacting the doctor or facility that submitted for payment as they may need to provide new or additional paperwork. Do not be surprised if mistakes take multiple calls and some time to correct, regardless of where the error occurred. *Sometimes* dealing with the insurance companies can feel like a full-time job. Some might consider it a really horrible full-time job. It helps to remind yourself that to them you are just another person paying premiums, and they are a business trying to hold on to their money for as long as possible. They don't care that you may not be feeling well. I found through this process the best line you can learn to use is, "help me understand…". For example: *"Please, help me understand why this bill has not been paid." "Please help me understand what I need to do to correct this." "Please help me understand why you are such a stupid idi . . .*whoops – ignore that one. Use "Help me understand" generously as it works amazingly well in many situations with everyone on your team, including your doctors. I learned that it worked will in so many situations, I still often use it to this day.

- **Bills Paid:** Once you have received a bill and have compared it with the corresponding EOB, you will need to pay it. File the bill, the EOB, and a copy of how you paid it (online through bill pay, copy of the check, a printed receipt from your credit card) together in your binder. If you are making payments on the bill or have made any other arrangements, make notes on the bill and file. Notes are always a good thing as they can assist you should there be a problem. **Take names, note dates, and add anything pertinent.** (I had a four-figure bill at a hospital — where they had lost record of my payment — and because I had all the documentation, they were eventually able to locate that the payment had been applied to another patient's account.) Notes not only help, but can often clarify things like write-offs or payment arrangements.

- When you begin to make appointments with the different doctors, facilities, and other providers you will utilize in the process of your diagnosis and treatment, it is very important that you ask the right questions when you are attempting to find out if these physicians and facilities participate with your insurance plan. (I had it occur where I asked a doctor's office if they accepted my insurance. They assured me that they did, indeed, accept my insurance. Not long after the visit I received a very large bill from this doctor and then the Explanation of Benefits, which explained that this doctor was NOT on my insurance (out of network), making me responsible for the entire billed amount. When I called the doctor's office to inquire about it, they told me they *accept* every insurance, but that they were not *__contracted__* with every insurance. You, as a patient, are required to pay 100% of all out-of-network expenses and the provider is NOT required to take any contracted write-off's, so providers are happy to "accept" your insurance.) Make sure as you begin to put your team together and begin the testing you will inevitably require, that you **SPECIFICALLY** ask them if they are *__CONTRACTED__* with your insurance company. Verbiage in this case truly matters!

- Review ALL your bills and compare them with the Explanation of Benefits. Especially review all hospital bills. It is not uncommon for there to be charges on a hospital bill for tests that were not performed or other items that should not have been included. If you see something on your bill that you are questioning, your first step is to contact the health care provider — hospital, doctor, facility — and communicate to them your dispute. If it is a hospital or surgical facility, you may need to request an itemized bill to compare them. (Most facilities only provide a complete breakdown of your bill, if requested.) If there is a test or service that you KNOW you did not have, ask them to provide a copy of the test results. That usually clears up the question of whether the test was completed or not. If the mistake is indeed genuine, you will need to ask the doctor or facility to re-submit an updated claim to your insurance company. You then want to contact the insurance company to let them know that there was a mistake in billing and that they should expect to be receiving an updated bill from the provider. You will want to make notes of the telephone number, date, time, who you spoke with, and if there are any confirmation numbers, codes, or any other specifics they can provide so that you have as much information as possible. This is important because many times after a bill has been submitted to your insurance company, and they have paid what **they** *think* is owed, it is not unusual for the insurance company to ignore resubmitted claims. Stay on top of this to hang on to as many of your hard-earned dollars as possible. Cancer is not an inexpensive diagnosis. I have saved LITERALLY *thousands* of dollars because insurance companies denied claims that were submitted with mistakes that I had corrected and resubmitted.

- ***DO NOT ignore your bills*** or Explanation of Benefits. Many companies have a time limit in which you can dispute a bill before you are obligated to pay it. If you miss this window to submit an appeal on a bill, you will be required to pay the entire amount, even if it is incorrect. As overwhelming as these bills can seem, being organized takes away much of the confusion and dread.

- If you are confused and don't understand your bill or the matching Explanation of Benefits, ask that doctor's billing department for assistance. Your doctor's office is aware of some of the challenges with the health insurance industry, so speaking with someone in the billing department can assist you in understanding your bill and support you in what is required to correct any errors. Doing this in person is often the most effective.

- Do not be surprised, especially if your cancer journey is a bit long, that dealing with insurance can sometimes feel like a full-time job. Often you are on hold for long periods of time and repeating the same information, several times, to several different people, even on the same call. That it is why it is so important to take as many notes as you possibly can and to get names of individuals when you are speaking with either your insurance company or a doctor's office about your bill. Also try to get a direct line number, as that may save time in the future when you can directly call the person handling your case.

- Once insurance has paid their portion and you have a large remaining balance, do not be afraid to pick up the telephone and ask the provider for a discount. (If the balance was applied to your deductible, you will **always** be required to pay that each year, no matter what.) Not everyone has the resources to pay, all at once, the large out-of-pocket expenses that could remain. There is nothing that stops you from trying to negotiate a lower out-of-pocket payment with the provider once insurance has paid their portion. You can ask the provider, *"Would you consider accepting what insurance has paid as payment in full?"* This tells them that you would like them to write off the remainder of the balance. They may not agree to that, but you might as well start by asking for it all to be written off and from there negotiate a discount. Some doctors have what they call a "No Insurance Rate," which is something they offer to patients with no insurance. It is often a much-reduced amount compared to the insurance rate. After your insurance has paid, contact your provider, and ask them if they have a "No Insurance Rate." Then ask them what that rate is for the services you had and compare the two fees. If your insurance company has already reimbursed your doctor the equivalent of the doctor's "No Insurance Rate," or even more, ask them if they would accept **that** amount as payment in full. That means that whatever your insurance paid is applied to the bill and then the bill is refigured, so you only pay whatever that remaining difference is for the "No Insurance Rate," if there is any. That could be the difference of several hundred dollars on just one bill. For example: you have a procedure that your insurance is billed $2000, your insurance reimburses your doctor $600 leaving a balance of $1400. If their "No Insurance Rate" is $1200, you could ask them if they would accept the $1200 as payment in full, thus saving you $200. (Many offices may not negotiate, but not asking will ALWAYS mean you pay the entire amount.

- If you are checking with your insurance company for insurance coverages for wigs, DO NOT ask if they cover "wigs" — ask instead if they cover a cranial prosthesis. This will be the insurance language that will get you coverage, if it is a part of your plan.

- Having a speaker phone or using the speaker feature on your cell phone is beneficial as it allows you to go about your business in case you are on hold for an extended period with your insurance company – which is often the case.

$$\bullet \bullet \bullet$$

My Story:

I was due for my annual mammogram, so my plan was to start there and then schedule an appointment with my primary care doctor for what I thought was an inflamed lymph node.

Wham, bam, mammogram.

For me, mammograms have never been any big deal. I have been having annual Smoosh My Breasticles since I turned 40, due to a positive family history of breast cancer, cysts that my doctor had been following for decades, and because I have very dense breasts. EVERYTHING felt lumpy on a simple self-exam or exams by my doctors. So, I have been having mammograms, or mammograms and ultrasounds, annually, for many years.

My plan was once it came back as normal, which I felt certain it would, I would go to my primary care physician. I wanted him to look at what was going on in my left armpit to see if I had anything that required treatment. An infection. A pulled muscle. I knew it was nothing serious, but it was annoying as hell and I was committed to being proactive about my health. It's my experience that many of us in the medical field are terrible patients and I, admittedly, am very guilty. I tend to let things drag on for quite some time before I do something about it. But for some reason I kept having this nagging feeling in my gut that I needed to have this checked out.

On 7/10/14 I went in for a routine 3D mammogram. A couple days later I received a call from the imaging facility that my results had come back suspicious and that they wanted to repeat the mammogram. They saw a minor cluster of calcium deposits in a very small spot. However, they suspected that it was either deodorant or perfume — even though I knew I had worn neither that day — so they wanted to repeat the exam. On 7/21/14 I had my second mammogram with the same results. There was a tiny (about the size of the head of a little nail) spot of calcification that the radiologist felt was more than likely just an age-related change, but he recommended a biopsy, as it had not shown up on any of my previous Smooshes.

(I credit this never-seen radiologist with saving my life. If he had missed this teeny weensy little speck of calcification, I may not be here to be writing this right now. No, I'm certain I WOULD NOT be here writing this today. He is one of the many unsung heroes that are often behind the scenes but are so valuable to the thing that is most important for all cancer patients...early detection. I even took the time to find his name and I wrote him a thank you note as it was no lost on me that without him picking up the small spot in a very dense breast, my stage 3 diagnosis could have become a metastatic diagnosis.)

A Guided Fine Needle Aspiration Biopsy (FNAB) was scheduled for July 30. I was more curious than nervous. I had spent 20 years in medicine for a reason. I like the blood, gore, and gaping wounds. I like being in surgery and opening organs. I like watching surgeries being performed and I love assisting in those surgeries. Emergencies make my heart palpitate with excitement wondering what might be coming through the door and guessing what we would be doing to treat it. I LOVE it! So, my own biopsy seemed trivial but worthy of the curiosity of what would be occurring. I was not concerned in the slightest.

As with many of the tests and procedures I've experienced in my life, I wasn't told what to expect. I didn't Google it online; I just showed up. What I wasn't expecting was to be lying face down on an elevated table with my breasticles dangling through a hole strategically located on the table. What did I think was going to happen? Today, looking back, I have no idea. I mean, I was told it was a biopsy. I guess I just hadn't really given it too much thought about how that might occur. I just wanted to get it over with, so the girls could get a clean bill of health. Then I could go find out why the hell my under arm annoyed me so much and get it fixed!

With my large left breast hanging through the hole in the elevated table, gently swaying in the breeze, the doctor and technician began to position me and tell me what to expect. After some moving around and repositioning, he could precisely pinpoint the spot and administered a local anesthetic. With me joking with them that if my breast hit the floor would they please not step on it and some other sassy, and probably, inappropriate things having to do with large, long, breasts he positioned me again and inserted a needle in the spot to remove a tissue sample.

About 25 minutes after my stomach hit the table, I was done. Numb in a small area from the anesthesia, but done. The technician had me sit upright for a few minutes, and while I got my sea legs back, the radiologist chatted with me for a few minutes. He reassured me that I really didn't have anything to worry about; it looked just like a little cluster of calcium, that these are usually age-related changes, and that less than 10 percent of these types of clusters come back as cancer. AND those few that do come back as cancer are almost always what is termed in situ, meaning the growth or tumor is still confined to the site where it started and that it is rarely an invasive type of cancer.

I left feeling more than optimistic. I wasn't even concerned. A little sore...but not at all apprehensive.

The day of the biopsy was a Wednesday. I was told the results could be as early as before the weekend. Woohoo. By Friday at 5 p.m. I had heard nothing. I'm a firm believer in that no news is good news and bad news travels fast. I was certain that since there hadn't been any urgent call, everything was fine, there was nothing to worry about and I spent the weekend hosting a Little League Baseball tournament.

Next step in the plan — make an appointment with my primary care physician.

DIAGNOSIS

More than 1 million people in the United States receive a cancer diagnosis each year. And lucky you (sarcasm font), you've been told that some lump, bump, mole, or blood test not only came back as suspicious, but you've heard the "C" word — CANCER. Other than a death in a family or of someone you love immensely, I'm not sure there is a scarier thing to hear than, "I'm sorry, but you have cancer."

CANCER, regardless of how soon it has been caught, generally is a scary diagnosis to hear. However, a diagnosis now is much better than a diagnosis even as little as five years ago, due to the advances that have been made in detection and treatment.

KNOWLEDGE IS POWER. The more you know, the more intelligent questions you can ask so that you really are a part of your own diagnosis, treatment, healing, and ultimately Survivorship. Knowledge is also empowering. That is the goal here: to hopefully not overwhelm you with too much information, and to give you enough to empower you as you progress through this diagnosis. **I will warn you** to not try to get much of your knowledge from the internet. Unless a website ends in .edu, .org, or .gov you should avoid researching your diagnosis online, especially if you have not received a full diagnosis yet. This often can lead you to forums and websites that are filled with misinformation, uneducated material, and disinformation. If I could tell you to avoid the internet at all costs, I would. But in an age when we carry little computers in our pockets, it's second nature to "Google" it. Again, just be careful of the resources you choose to get your information from.

DIAGNOSIS

A cancer diagnosis is *usually* **not** an emergency — although it sure feels like it. (When I was diagnosed all, I could think was get this uninvited guest out of me as quickly as possible! I don't have time for this!) Not only can it come completely as a surprise and often be overwhelming, it can also feel like a moving target as you move through the pathology and staging.

Two things will happen **FOR SURE** at the beginning of the diagnosis:

1) There will be an incredible flurry of activity as the doctor/s stage your cancer and decide upon a treatment plan.
2) You will endure what seems like an interminable amount of waiting.

These two things you can be assured of regardless of your situation.

• • •

What doctors are seeking to know before they formulate the best treatment strategy for you is:

- What kind of cancer do you have?
- How much cancer is in your body?
- Where is it located?
- What stage is the cancer?
- What grade is the cancer?
- Has it spread?

- What are the specific types of cells that make up the tumor?
- How aggressive is your cancer?

There are often several ways that a doctor can get this information, but it requires a pathologist (an expert who looks at cell or tissue samples under a microscope) to conduct laboratory testing to diagnose the cancer and to also determine answers to all those questions listed above.

A **biopsy** is usually the first step in determining if you actually have cancer and what type it is. The procedure takes out a piece of the lump, bump, or mole, which is then submitted to the **pathologist** for examination. Although there are some cancers that can be diagnosed without a biopsy, most cancers that have tumors require a biopsy of some sort.

• • •

Doctors also use other tests to look for cancer, to see if — or how far — it has spread and often to eventually determine if the treatment is working.

These tests can include:

- **X-Rays:** X-rays are good at showing bones and even some organs and soft tissues.

  - **Prep:** No special preparation is usually needed for an X-ray other than removing any metal objects you might have in your body like piercings. An X-ray technician usually performs this test.
  - You will typically be asked to undress to expose the part of the body that is being x-rayed; you may be given a robe or a drape to wear. Depending on where they are x-raying, you may be asked to stand, sit, or

lie down. The technician will leave the room during your x-ray. Your exposure time for an x-ray is usually less than a second. There might be multiple images taken from multiple angles.

o The entire procedure will take about 10 or 15 minutes depending on the number of x-rays done. You can resume normal activity after they are completed.

- **Needle Biopsy:** This procedure is used to obtain a sample of cells for a pathologist. A needle biopsy may be used to take tissue or fluid samples from breasts, muscles, bones, and other organs such as the liver, kidney, or lungs. A physician with a technician, or team of technicians, performs the needle biopsy.

  o **Prep:** Most needle biopsies do not require any preparation on your part, unless you are taking blood-thinning medications such as Coumadin, Plavix, or aspirin and some supplements like fish or coconut oils. If you are using any of these blood-thinning drugs or supplements, you may be instructed to stop them for a few days before the test, depending on what part of the body is being biopsied. You might also be instructed not to eat or drink before the procedure, especially if you are going to be receiving intravenous sedatives or general anesthesia for your biopsy.

  o After giving you a gown or drape, the technician/s will position you to make it easy for the doctor to access the spot where the needle will be inserted. Often an anesthetic will be injected into the skin around the area to make it numb. During the biopsy, the doctor guides a needle through your skin into the area of interest. This process may be repeated several times for the doctor to get enough cells or to biopsy multiple tumors. There are two common types of needle biopsies:

> **Fine-needle aspiration:** uses a thin, hollow needle to draw cells from your body.
> **Core needle biopsy:** uses a wider needle than a fine-needle aspiration. This larger needle allows the doctor to extract a core of tissue for testing.

o With most biopsies, a local anesthesia is used to numb the area. You may experience pressure or mild discomfort. Once the doctor has collected enough cells or tissue, your procedure is done, and your samples will be sent to the pathologist for analysis. The doctor or technician will place a bandage over the area where the needle was inserted. You may be asked to apply pressure for several minutes to decrease any bleeding.

o Usually, you can leave once your biopsy is completed, however, depending on where in your body the biopsy was performed, you may be asked to stay for a few hours while the medical team observes you to make sure you have no complications. Plan to take it easy for the rest of the day and keep the area covered for as long as you are instructed. You might feel some tenderness or discomfort in that area, but that usually resolves in a day or two. You may even have some bruising around or near the biopsy site, but that, as well, usually resolves in a few days.

• **CT Scan:** CT or CAT scans capture a cross section, or a slice, of the body, and show your bones, organs and soft tissues. These images show additional parts more clearly than just a regular X-ray. CT scans can show the size, shape, and location of cancer tumors. They can also show

40

blood vessels that may feed the tumor without having to put the patient through a surgical procedure.

- **Prep:** CT scans are most often done as an outpatient procedure. This may be at a hospital or an imaging facility where they have a CT scan machine. As with an X-ray, a technician will usually perform the test. The CT scanner is a large donut-shaped machine that has a flat table that slides back and forth inside the large donut hole. The scanner shoots beam through your body in order to create the image.
- Once you are in a gown or drape, the technician will leave the room for the test but will communicate with you via a microphone. You may be instructed to hold your breath for a short time and you will be asked to hold very still as movement can affect the image. A CT scan is usually painless, but you may find it a bit uncomfortable to hold yourself in a certain position for the minutes it takes to perform the test. Depending on the part of the body being scanned, you may need to drink a contrast liquid or have a contrast enema just prior to the testing. Sometimes your doctor will want a CT scan with an intravenous contrast dye. If you are having a scan with contrast, they will likely do a scan first and then do another after the contrast is given for comparison. You may experience a warm feeling throughout your body after the contrast is injected, but it is a brief and not uncomfortable feeling that goes away quite quickly. Some people also experience a bit of a metallic taste, which also subsides quickly.
- A CT scan can take anywhere from 10 to 30 minutes, but it may actually take much longer to position you for the test than the actual scan itself. You may also be asked to wait a few minutes after the test is completed while they check to make sure the images are clear. This is fairly routine; don't get nervous if

they do ask you to wait a few minutes, or even retake more images. After the scan, you can usually return to your normal activities, unless instructed otherwise.

- **MRI:** Magnetic Resonance Imaging also creates a cross-section of your body. MRIs assist doctors in finding cancer in the body and help them see if it has spread. It can also help doctors with their plan for cancer treatment.

  ○ **Prep:** You will usually be able to eat and drink as normal unless instructed otherwise.
  ○ Disclose any metal in your body such as surgical clips, staples, screws, plates, artificial joints, breast expanders, pacemakers, artificial heart valves, and infusion ports — basically, any metal in your body. These things may keep you from being able to have an MRI.
  ○ You will be asked to undress and be given a gown or drape. You will want to make sure you remove all metal earrings, piercings, or jewelry. You may also be asked to remove any non-permanent dental work like dentures. The machine is a long, narrow cylinder and your will lie down on a narrow, flat table. The technician will likely use straps, pillows or foam to make you as comfortable as possible and support you to stay in place. You will be in the room alone, but you will be able to speak with the technician throughout the test via a microphone. The test is painless, but you are inside a small cylinder. This means the surface of the machine might be quite close to your face. The machine makes loud thumping, clicking, and whining noises throughout the scan, so you will be given earplugs or headphones to muffle the noise. The noise and confined space may make some people anxious. If you think you might be one of those

people, you can ask the referring physician for some medication to take prior to the test to relax you, or you can investigate if there is an open MRI in your area. An open MRI may not produce images as clear or detailed as a closed MRI, and it may not be covered by your insurance company; you may just need to put on your big girl panties or big boy britches and just have the test. If you know you are going to be nervous, be sure to tell your doctor so he or she can provide you with the appropriate medications to relax you just prior to the test. (If you are given these medications, you **must** have a driver.)

o MRI scans usually take between 45 minutes to an hour, but sometimes can take as much as two hours, as this is another test that can be done with contrast. You may have to swallow the contrast, or it may be given intravenously. It is important to remain still during the testing and you may be instructed to hold your breath for a few seconds during the test. Do not be afraid to tell the technician if you need to move or take a break. After the test, you may be asked to wait a few minutes for the technician to confirm they have clear useful images. You can resume normal activity unless instructed otherwise.

- **Breast MRI:** Breast MRIs are mainly used for women who have already been diagnosed with breast cancer and are used to help measure the size of the tumor or to see if there are other tumors in the breast that may have been missed with mammography. This is especially important for women with dense breast tissue. Breast MRIs require a special MRI machine designed specifically for breast imaging. Not all hospitals or imaging facilities have these types of machines available, so you may be sent to a facility that is further away than a regular MRI facility. They must also be able to perform an MRI-guided breast biopsy, but the doctor who orders these tests will make sure you get to an appropriate facility that has dedicated breast MRI equipment.

- **Prep:** You will usually be able to eat and drink as normal unless instructed otherwise.
- You will need to take off clothes with metal parts such as zippers, snaps, or buttons. You will be given a gown or top. Like an MRI, if you have any metal in your body, you must let the technician know in advance. Some metal objects can cause problems, but others may be fine for this test. Just make sure you disclose to the technician any metal in your body or if you have breast tissue expanders or implants, if you are breastfeeding, or if you are possibly pregnant. For a breast MRI, you will have to lie face down on a specially designed platform inside a narrow tube. The platform has openings for each breast to hang through so they can be imaged without being compressed. The technician will likely use straps, pillows, or foam to make you as comfortable as possible. You will be in the room alone, but you will be able to speak with the technician throughout the test via a microphone. The machine makes loud thumping, clicking, and whining noises throughout the scan, so you will be given earplugs or headphones to muffle the noise. Some people are anxious about this. If you think you might be one of these people, you can ask your physician for some medication to take prior to the test to relax you. (If you get a relaxation medication, you **must** have a driver.) Unless your MRI is being done just as an evaluation, you will also have an IV with contrast to help identify the structures of the breast.
- Breast MRIs can often take up to an hour. Be sure to get as comfortable as you possibly can and to alert the technician before you move for any reason. You can

usually return to full activity after the test, unless instructed otherwise.

- **MRI-Guided Breast Biopsy:** This is similar to an MRI and is used when mammography or other imaging cannot tell if a growth is benign or cancerous. MRI-guided breast biopsies are performed by taking samples of the abnormality with MRI guidance.

  o **Prep:** You will usually be able to eat and drink as normal unless instructed otherwise.
  o You will need to take off clothes with metal parts such as zippers, snaps, or buttons. You will be given a gown or top. Like with an MRI, you will need to remove anything metal prior to the test, and if you have any metal in your body, you must let the technician know. Some metal objects can cause problems, but others may be fine for this test. Just make sure you disclose to the technician any metal in your body or if you have breast tissue expanders or implants, if you are breastfeeding, or if you are possibly pregnant. The technician will insert an IV for contrast if necessary. Like with the breast MRI, you will have to lie face down on a specially designed platform inside a narrow tube. The platform has openings for each breast to hang through in order to image them without compressing them. The technician will use straps, pillows, or foam to make you as comfortable as possible and better support you in position. Then a local anesthetic will be injected into the breast by a specially trained breast radiologist to numb the area so a very small incision can be made in the skin where the biopsy needle is inserted. The radiologist then inserts the needle and advances it to the location of the tumor. After the tissue sample or samples have been excised, the needle will be removed. A small marker will be placed

at the site of the biopsy so that its specific area can be located in the future by your surgeon or radiologist.

o This guided biopsy usually takes about 45 minutes. Once the procedure is completed, the technician will apply pressure to stop any bleeding and you may get small Steri-strips or the site may be covered with only a bandage. Sutures are usually not necessary. You are often a bit sore after this procedure and it is not unusual to feel a lump at the site of the biopsy or to have bruising that may last several days. You can usually return to your normal activity unless instructed otherwise. This test can also make you a bit nervous. If you think that will be you, be sure to let your doctor know so they can prescribe medication to relax you prior to the biopsy. However, if you use medication to relax you, you **must** have a driver.

- **Angiogram:** This test is used to look at arteries in the body including the brain, lungs, and kidneys. It can be done with X-rays and/or a CT Scan.

  o **Prep:** An angiogram can be done by different types of doctors, including a radiologist, cardiologist, or surgeon. You will most likely be asked not to eat before this test, and you will probably be given medicine to relax you before the test starts. You will be on a table where you will be asked to lie still. With CT angiography the contrast dye will usually go into a small vein through an IV in the arm. A tiny cut will be made so the plastic tube (catheter) can be put into a blood vessel — usually in the artery at the top of the thigh — and slid in until it reaches the area to be evaluated. The contrast dye is injected, and a series of X-ray pictures are done to see how the dye goes through the vessels.

o Pressure will be applied to the site after the catheter is removed. You will be moved to another, more comfortable table, where you will also have to lie flat and keep your leg still for several hours to prevent bleeding where the catheter was inserted in your leg. Because of the need to make sure you have no active bleeding after the exam, this test and the post-test recovery can take several hours. You will require a driver. You will be given instructions after the test is complete about your post-test activities.

- **Intravenous Pyelogram (IVP):** This test is used to study your urinary tract — including kidneys, ureters, and bladder — and is usually done on an outpatient basis by a specially trained technician.

  o **Prep:** You will probably be instructed not to eat or drink anything for about 12 hours before the test and you will be given instructions on how to use laxatives to clean out your bowels. For the test, you will be on an x-ray table where you will have a series of x-rays done. Then, through an IV, you will receive contrast dye. Another series of x-rays is taken over the next 30 minutes to get images of the dye as it moves through your kidneys and out of your body. There may be slight pressure applied to your abdomen to help make the images clearer. Once the contrast has reached your bladder, you will be asked to urinate while another x-ray is taken.
  o An IVP is usually completed within an hour; however, because some kidneys function at a slower rate, the exam may last up to four hours. You can return to normal activity after this test.

- **Lower GI Series:** This test is used to check your colon and rectum, and it is done in a hospital or outpatient facility. This examination is done by a specially trained doctor.

- ○ **Prep:** You will be instructed about your diet for the few days before the test. There are often restrictions in what you can eat prior to the test. You will also be given laxatives to clean out your bowels. You will not be given anesthesia for this exam. For the test, you will be strapped to a special table and a series of x-rays will be taken. Once those are finished, liquid barium is put into your bowels through a small tube inserted in your rectum. More images will be taken while the table is tilted or while you are instructed to move into different positions for more images. This will move the barium through your bowels so the bowels can be seen on the x-rays. You must lie still, and you will be instructed to hold your breath as each image is taken.
- ○ A lower GI usually takes 30 to 60 minutes. After the test, you will be told to go to the restroom to pass the barium. It may take a few days for it all to evacuate, and you may notice that your stool is drier, lighter colored, and even harder until all the barium is out of your body. You may have some cramping and bloating after the procedure. You can resume most normal activities after the procedure is completed. You must arrange to have a driver.

- **Upper GI Series:** This test is utilized to look at your esophagus, stomach, and small intestine, and it is done in a hospital or outpatient facility. This test is done by a specially trained doctor and an x-ray technician.

  - ○ **Prep:** You will likely be instructed not to eat or drink anything for about 12 hours before this test. You will not need anesthesia. Much like the lower GI series, you will be asked to sit or stand in front of an x-ray machine while a series of X-rays are done after you have swallowed the barium mixture, or you will be asked to lie on an x-ray table while the radiologist watches the barium move through the GI tract. You will be asked to swallow some throughout the test and you may be asked to swallow other substances as well.

○ This test usually takes about two hours, but you may be asked to remain, or return a few hours later, for additional X-rays that will look at the small intestines. It takes time for the barium to arrive there, so this test could take a total of five hours. You will be given a laxative after the test to speed up the removal of the barium from your body, but you can expect that your stool may be drier, lighter in color, and harder until the barium is gone. You will be given instructions after the test and you will want to follow them closely. You should not need a driver.

- **Colonoscopy:** (or a Sigmoidoscopy) This test allows the doctor to look at the inside of the entire colon and rectum (or part of the colon and rectum if it is a sigmoidoscopy.) It is performed by a specially trained doctor in a hospital or outpatient facility.

  ○ **Prep:** You will do what is known as a bowel prep and it is usually the worst part of these two tests. You might be told to avoid certain foods and medicines a few days before the test, as they may have dyes in them that can impact the test results. You will get instructions from your doctor ahead of time regarding the need for a clear liquid diet for 24 hours before your procedure, as well as instructions about taking strong laxatives to clean out your colon before the procedure.

  ○ The actual procedure takes about 30 minutes and is performed by a doctor. However, you will usually be instructed to arrive earlier than your test time as they will start an IV to help you relax and/or to sleep for a brief period while the test is being performed. You are usually there for two to three hours and you **must** have a driver as you cannot drive for 24 hours after this procedure. Your doctor will give you instructions about resuming your normal diet and activities.

- **Endoscopy:** This test is done by a specially trained doctor who uses a long, flexible tube with a camera, to see the lining of your upper GI tract. This test is usually done in a hospital, outpatient facility, or even some doctors' offices and is usually done under light anesthesia.

  - **PREP:** To make sure the GI tract is clear for this test, your doctor will advise you not to eat, drink, smoke, or chew gum during the eight hours before the test. Your doctor will also instruct you on any medications you must discontinue prior to the exam. You will most likely be given an IV sedative, but sometimes this test is done without sedation and you are given a liquid anesthetic to gargle instead. You will be asked to lie on your side on the table while the doctor feeds the camera down your esophagus and into your stomach.
  - The procedure generally takes about 15 to 30 minutes, but you are usually there a couple of hours because of the anesthesia. You may experience some bloating and a sore throat for a day or two. You **must** have a driver. Your doctor will give you instructions about resuming your normal diet and activities.

- **PET Scan (Positron Emission Tomography):** This test allows the doctor to see if the cancer may have spread to other parts of your body. It can show cancer in the lungs, bones, liver, adrenal glands, and other organs. (It may also be utilized to tell if certain treatments are working.)

- **PREP:** This test is usually done as an outpatient procedure, and is performed by a technician using a form of radioactive sugar known as a tracer. You are usually given specific instructions prior to the test, which vary depending on the type of PET scan you are having. You will likely be asked not to drink any sugary liquids of any kind for several hours before the test and you may also be asked not to eat anything for several hours prior to the test. You may be given a gown to wear or you may be allowed to wear your own clothing. Depending on the type of scan you are having done, the radioactive tracer is either given in your vein, given to be swallowed, or it is inhaled as a gas. This sugar binds to cells in your body. Cells that are growing rapidly, such as cancer cells, will take up larger amounts of sugar than normal cells, which shows up on the PET scan. (Some doctors will combine a PET scan with a CT scan, which might show more detail in certain areas and give the doctor more information to pinpoint tumors more precisely.) It typically takes 60 minutes for the tracer to travel through your body and to be absorbed by the tissue and organs being studied. You will be asked to sit and rest quietly, avoiding movement, talking, reading, or watching television. After the hour, you will be moved to the scanner. The PET scanner is a large machine with a round, donut-shaped hole, very much like a CT scan or MRI.
- The scanning time is usually about 30 minutes; however, depending on which organ or tissue is being examined, you may have additional tests involving other tracers, which could lengthen the procedure time to three hours. When the scan is completed, you may be asked to wait while the technician checks the

results to make sure no additional images are required. Through the natural process of radioactive decay, the tracer in your body will lose its

- o radioactivity over time. It will also pass out of your body through your urine and stool following the test, so you will want to be diligent with washing your hands for the next couple days. You should drink plenty of fluids to help flush the tracer out of your body and you might be told not to hold children or pets in your lap for a short period of time. Unless you have been told otherwise, you should be able to return to normal activity after a PET scan; however, if any special instructions are necessary, the technician will inform you.

- **Bone Scan:** A bone scan is a nuclear medicine test that can be used to find out if the cancer has started in or spread to the bones. Bone scans can also be used to see how well treatment is working.

  - o **Prep:** A specifically trained technologist will perform this test either in a nuclear medicine department of a hospital or an outpatient imaging center. There is usually no special preparation for this test. You will be given a tracer through a vein in your arm; you will not feel the tracer as it moves through your body. It takes anywhere from one to four hours for your bones to absorb the tracer. After the waiting period, you will lie on your back on an exam table. During the scan the camera will move slowly around your body. You will need to lie still during the test; however, the technician may ask you to change positions to get images from a different angle. A whole-body scan takes about an hour to complete. You will want to drink water after your test to remove the radioactive material that has not collected in your bones.

These are just some of the diagnostic tests for cancer, and many of them will not apply to your current situation. (Also, depending on what country you live in or what year you are reading this, there are any number of different and new tests that are making it easier to detect and treat cancer sooner. Yay!)

It is after any number of these tests that your team will begin to take shape. These tests will tell your doctor what type of cancer you have and what you require to treat it. Do you need a surgeon, radiation oncologist, or medical oncologist? Or perhaps your type of cancer has you lucky enough to require only being followed by tests each year? Once your doctor has the results of these tests, they will refer you to the appropriate specialists and will begin to put together their recommendation for you. Often there are multiple options and you will have an opportunity to collaborate with your cancer team to determine the best treatment option/s for you given your type of cancer, stage, prognosis, age, and other factors. Just know that your team will have the best approach for you when they give you their recommendations.

• • •

Tips:

- Always double check that your **procedure** is covered by your insurance. Almost all insurance companies require prior authorization for diagnostic testing. Make sure that the doctor that orders the test takes care of all the required precertification to have the test covered by your insurance.
- Make sure that the **facility** where the procedure is going to be performed is covered by your insurance. Often a

doctor has privileges at a facility that he prefers, but that facility may not be **contracted** with your insurance.

- Be sure to ask if other doctors are going to be involved. For example: you may go in for a colonoscopy and that simple procedure also involves an anesthesiologist, who will sedate you, and the pathologist, who will read the slides of the biopsy. If there are others involved, make sure **THOSE** doctors are **contracted** with your insurance, prior to the procedure. Making sure that all the doctors involved are **contracted** with your insurance may slow the process, as the scheduling assistant may have to do additional work to assure they are all available. It is worth being patient as it may mean the difference between you paying *NOTHING* out of pocket or you paying *SEVERAL thousands of dollars.*

- Always ask how much time you should *set aside for a test*. I once made the mistake of asking how long the test would take and I was told less than an hour. What they failed to tell me was that everything leading up to the test, and how long they needed to watch me after completion of the test required that I actually be there for three hours. Ask *how long you will be there*, not how long the test takes. Many tests don't take long at all, but the prep, set-up, and recovery can take several hours.

- If the facility doesn't call a day or two prior to the procedure, be sure to contact them. This may save you some time completing paperwork, as some facilities will fax or email the admission paperwork to you and/or go over it via the telephone. You will also want to confirm, at that time, that everything has been prior-authorized ("prior auth" in medical office jargon) and that all the doctors are **contracted** with your plan. Ask if they have any confirmation numbers they can provide and be sure to add those notes to your three-ring binder for future reference, if necessary.

...

My Story:

Remember I mentioned having just enough medical knowledge to make me a pain in the ass? Well, I use that perceived knowledge when I attend doctor appointments with Mom and my in-laws. My in-laws are in their 90's and my mom, who is confined to a wheelchair, is in her 80's. I consider it an honor to be their patient advocate — an honor that they would trust me enough to be there on their behalf and to know I will ask questions that because of my healthcare experience, they may not even have thought of. Having a little bit of medical knowledge, although a pain in the ass to most doctors, is most useful when you are a patient advocate to your family.

The Monday following my biopsy, August 4, was one of those days for my "Patient Advocate" hat. My father-in-law (I call him FIL) had been having heart problems and shortness of breath for several weeks and had been scheduled for a Pulmonary Function Test at a hospital across town. I was to be at his house at 6:30 a.m. to have him at the hospital for the test at 7:00.

The appointment became one of those times where the scheduling procedure broke down and ultimately failed. We arrived on time for the test, yet they had no orders from his doctor's office. To top it off, it was two hours before the doctor's office would open. The admitting office suggested we wait and they would contact the on-call doctor to see if he had any knowledge about the test. After waiting for over an hour to hear back, the on-call doctor said he had no idea what test was supposed to have been ordered to be performed since he wasn't FIL's regular doctor. They suggested we return home and figure it out when the referring doctor's office opened.

Feeling incredibly frustrated (FIL had not been feeling well for weeks and this appointment was supposed to give us the definitive results), I was taking him back to his house when my phone rang. I typically don't answer my phone when I'm driving, but seeing it was my Vaginacologist, who, for the 30 years I have been her patient, has always called me with my test results, I decided to answer it rather than jump through the hoops of trying to return her call.

The conversation went pretty much like this:

Me: Hello, Dr. J.
Dr.: Hello.
Me: How are the girls? (Our two children were the same ages, so I always asked about her girls.)
Dr.: They're good. I'm here in my office and I'm going over the lab results that came in over the weekend and I have your biopsy results in front of me.
Me: That's great.
Dr.: Well, it's actually not so great.
Me: Okaaaaay??
Dr.: Your biopsy shows you have breast cancer.
Me: Okaaaaay??
Dr.: And surprisingly it isn't as we would have expected — in situ — it shows it is an invasive breast cancer.

*At **that** moment, I knew three things were happening simultaneously:*

1) *I was driving my car down 19th Avenue in Phoenix, Arizona, with FIL.*
2) *I was on the phone with my doctor who had just told me I had cancer.*
3) *All the sudden I was no longer in my own body. It was as if I were suddenly watching everything take place from the headliner of my vehicle.*

56

Care Team Selection

As your tests results come back you will begin to put together your team of specialists. There are several ways to find a doctor who specializes in your type of cancer:

- Primary care referral
- Local Hospital
- National Institute for Cancer
- American Medical Association
- American Society of Clinical Oncology
- American College of Surgeons
- Facebook. (Don't laugh. It seems like everyone has either had cancer themselves or knows someone who has had cancer. I was stunned by the number of my friends that, when they learned about my diagnosis, told me about themselves, their sibling, their parent, or even their friends that had cancer. Some of us even used the same physicians.) If you don't want to go public on Facebook, you can always ask for a "friend" or have a trusted friend ask for you.

However, regardless of whom you have been referred to, your insurance will dictate who you can see. Unless you are blessed with such abundant resources that your insurance coverage limits do not matter, you will quite possibly need to get **several** referrals to specialists in order to find one that is

CONTRACTED with your insurance AND is accepting new patients.

• • •

There are three main types of cancer treatments in the United State, as of this writing, but many different and even less invasive treatments are becoming available all the time. But for now, the three main types of conventional treatment are:

- Surgery
- Radiation
- Chemotherapy

Depending on your diagnosis, you may need to be referred to a radiation oncologist; or perhaps a radiation oncologist and a surgeon; or you might have won the cancer trifecta and you get to share your experience with all three — a radiation oncologist, a surgeon, and a medical oncologist.

My surgeon explained it to me in a way I could easily understand by telling me that surgery takes care of the tumor, radiation takes care of the cells surrounding the tumor, and chemotherapy takes care of any of the little bastards that have gotten away and are floating around your body, only to hang around and eventually wreak havoc all over again. (Okay, he didn't say that, but it's pretty much how that obnoxious little voice in my head translated it.)

I was referred to my surgeon first and he recommended, and referred me to, my other doctors as my diagnosis evolved. His office also made sure that each doctor he was referring me to was **CONTRACTED** with my insurance plan before sending me there.

(Side Note: There are currently other cancer treatments as well — immunotherapy, targeted cancer therapies, hormone therapy, stem cell transplant, and, depending on when and where you are reading this, I hope many, many more. Some are still investigational; some are in clinical trial phases; some are currently available and being utilized as first-line therapy. There are also clinical trials available that you might be a candidate for. In addition, there are naturopathic oncology groups around the country. However, I'm going to speak to current conventional therapy — surgery, radiation, and chemotherapy.)

Not only should you get several names of doctors to make sure you find ones **CONTRACTED** with your insurance company, I also recommend you have multiple choices as you may not feel comfortable with the first physician you meet.

It is so very important to have a comfortable relationship with your doctor. How well you can communicate with this person (and they are ONLY people) is an essential part of getting the care that is best for YOU. If you meet a doctor for the first time and don't feel comfortable with them, do not hesitate to interview another. You really are "interviewing" these physicians. You do not have to choose the very first one you go to. (I personally know someone who interviewed four surgeons before she found the one she felt comfortable with.)

It may not have gone *exactly* this way, but when I met my surgeon, I recall it going something like:

"Hi, I'm Dr. Breast Surgeon and you and I are about to become best friends."

It really will be like that. You are going to be spending a lot of time with this person, possibly showing them parts of your body that you reserved showing to only those closest to you. (Or maybe no one at all. My internal organs used to be off limits to anyone!) You may be having conversations about bowel movements, vomiting, drainage, pain, sutures, funny little things that start happening to your body that you may think is nothing, but in your treatment, could actually be something very important. You may even need to talk about...............sex. (EEEK!) So, it's best to feel comfortable enough to be able to discuss everything. You need to feel like they are your best friend and that you are so comfortable with them that you could tell them anything.

Sometimes, like a marriage, you think you picked "the one" and you find that as you go along you start to have challenges. Usually, like marriage, it is just a communication issue and there are ways to make it healthier. It is best to try and work it out before deciding to "divorce" them.

To work it out, you must be open and honest with your doctor.

Here are some things you can say to start a difficult conversation:

- *"I'm having trouble understanding_____. Can you help me understand?"*
- *"I feel like we aren't communicating well, and here's why..."*
- *"I realize you are busy and sometimes I feel too rushed to discuss_____ with you. Can we schedule a time to do that?"*
- *"I need to talk with you about_____, but feel like I can't. Can we discuss this?"*

However, you may be like me; I would do *anything* to avoid a confrontation. This is when it is nice to have someone along as your advocate. Enroll someone who you trust, explain to them your challenge, and let them convey it to the doctor. Here are some examples:

- Your friend could say for you, "My friend tells me that she is having trouble understanding_____. Can you help me help her understand?"
- Your spouse could say for you, "My wife tells me she doesn't feel like you two are communicating well, and here's why."
- As a parent you could say, "Doctor, I realize you are busy, but sometimes my daughter feels you are too rushed to discuss _____. Can we schedule a time to do that?
- If you are supporting a sibling, "Doctor, my sister was sharing with me that she feels like she can't talk with you about_____. Would you go over that with us?"

Sometimes, like marriage, you've tried it all and you realize (or perhaps you both realize) it's time to say enough is enough. Don't stay with a doctor because you are worried about hurting their feelings. Just because you were referred to that doctor doesn't mean it is always going to be a match made in heaven or that you shouldn't find a new doctor. It's your cancer journey now, and DAMMIT, you have the right to choose the best doctor for you!

If you choose to find a different doctor, be sure to ask for all of your records and their office notes be copied for you to take to your new doctor.

• • •

Tips:

- Be honest with your doctor about your habits, like drinking or smoking, even if you aren't proud of them. Quite frankly your doctor is busy treating your cancer;

they are not going to judge your drinking, drug use, or smoking. But it is imperative information for them to have in order to make sure you get the appropriate care and possible drug interactions are avoided.

- Do not be afraid to tell your doctor how much you do or don't want to know. Personally, I want all the details (and pictures and diagrams if you got 'em.) But experience tells me I am in the minority. Some people want to know **nothing**. (I've met survivors that didn't even know what kind of cancer they had. They didn't want any specifics. They just wanted to be told what to do.) I think most people are somewhere in the middle. Just be sure and let your doctor know where that is for you.

- Take someone to all your appointments; especially when you are seeing a doctor for the first time. It is not unusual to be anxious and afraid, which makes it hard to concentrate. Another pair of ears (or several pairs) is the best solution.

- If you are a private person and insist on not taking someone with you (I don't recommend it though!), ask the doctor if you can record the conversation. You can record from your smartphone or a recording device. You will want to explain to the doctor that, with their permission, you would like to record the examination and conversation, so you can refer to it in the future. (I will share that, personally, if I was interviewing a doctor and they voiced a hesitancy about that request, I would leave the appointment. If my doctor isn't comfortable enough with what they are saying and doing to be recorded, then I'm not comfortable enough with them treating me. But that's just me.)

- Carry a notebook with you everywhere. In the beginning, I would think of questions when I was out and about, then forget to write them down and promptly forget the question. Have a notebook handy to write things down so you won't forget.

- Use a notebook to take notes during appointments. (I then rewrote them in an orderly fashion in my "Notes" section of my three-ring binder; mainly because I can barely read my own handwriting so I wanted to transfer it so it was legible which also helped me to remember what was said and process it.)
- Take your three-ring binder to ALL your doctor appointments.
- Make sure you understand any instructions you've been given before you leave an appointment. Some tests and blood work may require you to fast; some tests require early arrival; sometimes you are told to just wait for a call back. It's easier to review the instructions and ask any questions before you leave the office. If I forgot to ask something and had to call the office, it often took a long time to get a response. (I know! I found it hard to believe that I wasn't their ONLY patient they were treating. They weren't just sitting around thinking of ways to cure me or waiting for me to call. The audacity! They actually had OTHER patients as well!) It's best to make sure you are clear about all directions before you leave the appointment.
- If you are unclear about something, do not hesitate to ask for clarification. If you are still unclear, ask your question in a different way. There is nothing wrong with telling your doctor that you don't understand. They do this cancer thing EVERY SINGLE DAY, with MANY patients and sometimes it can be forgotten that we are cancer neophytes. "Help me understand" is a phrase that comes in handy in these situations.
- If you want to know more about your cancer and they don't give you some material at the end of your visit, ask your doctor for suggested reading material or resources. It seems like every one of my doctors had pre-printed pamphlets, materials, or guides to give me. They may also have some preferred books to recommend, as well.

- I LOVE and HATE the internet for cancer information. There are many good resources for information. The best of them usually end with .org, .gov or .edu. If a website address ends with .com, be aware that it may not always be your best internet source for ACCURATE information. I also recommend you avoid most forums related to your cancer. These are often filled with misinformation or personal opinion. Take any information you get on web forums with a grain of salt. And if anyone in those forums suggests any kind of non-traditional therapies to you, be sure to run them by your doctor **before you try them.** Some recommendations are not problematic to try as adjunct therapy; however, there are some things that people recommend that might need to be avoided during your specific treatment or prior to surgery because of possible interatctions. Just be sure to ask your doctor **before** trying something new that was suggested to you or that you discovered online.
- Tell your physician about any vitamins or supplements you are currently taking. Some can have a negative impact on your treatment, while others may be just fine, or even recommended. Note them in your three-ring binder as if they are medications and make sure your care team knows about any new supplements you start.
- Find out where to call or what to do in case of an emergency.

• • •

My Story:

*After the shattering phone call with my doctor, I continued driving, still hovering somewhere outside of my body, and honestly so shocked, I can still, to this day, relive **that** moment* *and have all those same feelings. It was just so unreal; and at that moment, it felt as if it was happening to someone else.*

We didn't drive too much farther before FIL inquired:

"I heard you say you needed to go see a doctor. . . are you okay?"

[This is where that little lunatic voice in my head that never shuts up started yelling! Screaming! HELL NO! She's not okay!!!]

Me: "Well. . ."

[Don't tell him. It's all a big mistake!]

Me: ". . . I had two abnormal mammograms last month and last week I had to have a biopsy of a suspicious spot. My doctor received the results and she says I have breast cancer".

[SHUT! UP! LISTEN TO ME! It's all a mistake! Oh, for God's sakes now you've done it. You've actually said the "C" word. SHUT UP! SHUT UP!]

FIL: "Oh."

Me: "Uhm . . . yeah. She says it's small and they found it quite early, so I'm very lucky. She has given me a surgeon's name and she thinks it will just be a minor surgery and a few days of radiation, so it should all be fine."

FIL: (silence)

Me: "You can tell MIL (mother-in-law) but I would prefer you not say anything to anyone else until I've had a chance to tell your son. After that I'll decide to tell the kids or not."

[Tell the kids??? You aren't telling anyone!]

FIL: "I understand. Mum is the word until you tell me otherwise."

Still outside of my body, I dropped him off at his house and headed home. Home? Even that didn't seem real anymore. Nothing seemed real. My world was so off axis that I actually just wanted to keep driving and never stop.

The only good news was that it was found early and would be easy to treat. That's what made me head home rather than someplace — like a beach or a bar — to contemplate what I had just been told.

However, by the time I got home, I was even more out of my body. Nothing seemed real. Everything seemed to be moving in slow motion and the little voice in my head was blabbering so much, my head was about to explode.

How was this possible?

I had a busy life. I didn't have time for cancer.

I remember my calendar: 6:00 a.m. — leave house, 6:30 — pick up FIL, 7:00 — drive to the hospital. Call Pam and wish her happy birthday. NOWHERE did I see a damn thing about "have cancer."

This just could not be happening. I don't have time for this!

[WHAT. THE. ACTUAL.HELL?!!]

Hubby and I have a business together and he happened to be at our World Headquarters — our little home office — when I arrived back home. I shared with him the debacle with FIL's appointment. Hubby was as frustrated as I was, as this had been an ongoing concern with his father and we had been assured that the test results from that day would give us some insight on what was going on with him.

Then I said to him, "Dr. Vaginacologist called me with the results of the biopsy. It came back as breast cancer."

I recounted all she had said about it being small and early, and we again congratulated ourselves on being the "Lucky Lows."

Although it felt better to have told another person, I was still outside of my body, kind of watching everything take place, in slow motion, from what seemed like a million miles away. I could tell that Hubby was concerned; nonetheless he is a very optimistic person and when he said, "Hey, we've got this!" even though I was hearing it from miles away, I felt like, "Yeah, we do!"

Since it was still early in the morning, I called Dr. Breast Surgeon's office to schedule an appointment. He was, indeed, contracted with my insurance and figuring that it would take some time to get in, I was reeling when they said they could see me on Wednesday, just two days away! I almost wanted it to be a few days further away as I had the hope that I would get the call from Dr. Vaginacologist that it was all a big mistake.

I have several friends who have had the misfortune of having had breast cancer before me. One of these, Weezer, is someone that Hubby worked with for nearly 30 years. We are close. When SHE went through chemo, Hubby and our son, John, shaved their heads in support and stayed bald for as long as she was bald. I recalled that she had had a very negative first experience with a surgeon and I thought, based upon what she had been through, she would be a great person to go with me to get a feel for this recommended surgeon. I'm an unusually good judge of individuals, and my first impressions of people are usually dead on. Normally, I would have had no problem going by myself, but at that moment I felt anything but normal. And I knew that Hubby would feel more comfortable if she went with me, given how close they were, so I called her.

Fortunately, Weezer was available the day of the appointment to meet me at his office. Even with my years of medical background, this was all new territory and I wasn't trusting myself too much, yet, as a cancer patient. It was still too new, but I was so grateful she was available.

Now I just needed to make it through the next two days.

Selecting a Surgeon (Draft Day)

Since I had been a volunteer with Little League Baseball and Softball for so many years, I equate a lot of things in my life with baseball terminology. When I was referred to see Dr. Breast Surgeon, I started looking at it like a baseball game and putting together my team of players. There are so many baseball metaphors, analogies, and idioms that seemed to fit what I was getting ready to face. I saw myself as a "rookie batter," in the "top of the first inning," who had "stepped up to the plate" for the first time. The pitcher, Dr. Vaginacologist, had thrown me a first pitch "curveball" to the catcher, Dr. Breast Surgeon.

Catchers are considered the most important player on the field. Catchers are like a manager located on the field. Why? Communication. The key to any good relationship is communication, and catchers talk to coaches every inning, know exactly what is going on with all the other players, often direct and coach them, and are responsible for settling pitchers down when things may not be going smoothly.

Thus, my baseball debut began with me interviewing my potential catcher – The Surgeon.

When you are interviewing your team, you want to be prepared. If you are even remotely like me, you want to get answers. But how do you get answers when you don't even know the questions?

What I knew when I went to meet Dr. Breast Surgeon was that I had a small spot of cancer. At this point, it was only speculation on the part of Dr. Vaginacologist as to what they were going to do, but it would probably require surgery, and likely, radiation.

Cancer surgery, at this date, remains the foundation of cancer treatment. Your surgeon may use surgery for any number of reasons: from preventing and diagnosing cancer, to staging and treating it. One surgery is sometimes performed to take care of one, or more, of these things. And sometimes different surgeries may be required over a period of time to take care of preventing, diagnosing, staging, or treating your cancer.

You should always make sure that you get all of your questions answered when you are interviewing your surgeon. Here are some suggested questions (or they can be downloaded at www.holycrapihavecancer.com) you can utilize during your appointment. Keep in mind that some of these questions might seem premature, as occasionally surgery is utilized to stage your cancer, or some of the pathology reports may not have been completed yet. But utilize the questions that pertain to your particular situation, and be sure to add your own. You want to get as many of your questions answered as early in this process as you can so that you can stay empowered on this journey and can start processing and planning your next few weeks or months.

> - What is my diagnosis?
> - What Stage is my cancer?
> - What are my treatment options? What are the benefits of each option? What are the side effects?
> - Should I undergo genetic testing?
> - Will I need any additional testing?
> - What is the testing for?
> - What will the results of the additional testing tell you?
> - When will you get the results? How will I be informed?

- Why do I need surgery?
- What is the goal of this surgery: to take out the cancer, to remove some of the tumor to test for cancer, or to help with a problem the tumor is causing?
- What are the benefits?
- What are the chances it will work?
- How often is this surgery performed for my type of cancer?
- How many times have you done this procedure?
- What is your success rate?
- What are the possible complications, risks, or side effects?
- Why do I need this treatment?
- Do I have cancer in my lymph nodes?
- What is the significance of cancer found in the lymph nodes?
- Are there any other alternatives to treat the cancer or relieve the problem?
- Will I need other cancer treatments, like chemotherapy or radiation? Before or after surgery?
- What will happen if I don't have the operation?
- What do I have to lose or gain if I don't have this surgery?
- Am I healthy enough to have the surgery?
- Are you certified by the American Board of Surgery and/or a Specialty Surgery Board?
- Exactly what will you be doing during this surgery? What will you be removing and why?
- Will the surgery cure the cancer?
- How long will the surgery take?
- Who will update my family during surgery?
- Will I need blood transfusions?
- Do I need to do anything special to prepare for surgery?
- Will I have to stay in the hospital? If so, how long?
- What happens if the surgery doesn't work?
- What can I expect after surgery? Will there be a lot of pain? Will I have any drains or catheters coming out of my body?

- Can I sleep on my back, side, stomach?
- How soon can I shower after surgery?
- Do I have any restrictions and, if so, what are they and for how long?
- How will my body be affected by the surgery? Will it look or work differently? Will any of the changes be permanent?
- Will I be taking medicine after the surgery? How do you spell it? How will I take it?
- Are there any side effects?
- Will this medicine be okay to take with my other medications?
- How soon can I go back to work?
- Do I need to change my daily routine?
- How long before I can go back to my usual activities, like the gym?
- What about sex?
- Do I have time to think about the other options or get a second opinion?
- How quickly must I decide about my treatment?
- Will a delay in treatment reduce my chance of being cured?
- If I choose surveillance (monitoring or watching the cancer), or the cancer comes back, how will I be treated?
- What number should I call in an emergency?
- What is the name of the person I should communicate with in your office? Do they have a direct number?

These last two questions are usually addressed with the person responsible for billing:

- Will my insurance pay for this surgery?
- How much will my portion be?

You should never leave the surgeon's appointment with unanswered questions, unless they are about tests or pathology results that have not yet been completed.

• • •

Tips:

- Take your three-ring binder.
- Take someone with you and/or record the visit.
- Make a copy of the above questions to take with you. Cross out ahead of time all the questions you already know the answer to, or that are not pertinent to you, so that you can skip right over those.
- Make your notes on the question sheet you have copied.
- Transfer the answers to the copy in your three-ring binder.
- It is best that you not begin asking questions until your doctor is finished explaining what they know and then asks if you have any questions. Most doctors cover most of these questions as they explain your situation. If, at the end, they don't ask if you have questions, when it seems like they have covered everything, let them know you have a few questions. Keep this sheet handy and review each and every question, until you feel ALL of your questions have been answered.
- Remember that this is an interview with the person that now has your life in their hands. Treat it like that.
- Follow your gut!
- During follow-up visits ask what movements you can do to improve your range of motion and to decrease scarring. Movement is important to healing and recovery, but sometimes we are still experiencing discomfort, so we worry we might hurt something. Moving as quickly as your surgeon releases you will positively benefit your long-term recovery and reduces scarring and adhesions.

- Exercise makes a difference. Ask when you can begin to exercise (even if it is just a short 10-minute stroll) or when you can return to your normal exercise routine.

• • •

My Story:

I wouldn't say that it was love at first site when I met Dr. Breast Surgeon, but it was pretty close. There was a calm demeanor about him that put me at ease from the second he walked in the exam room. Together we looked at my mammogram results and he, in great detail, explained my options. He explained that the pathology from my biopsy was still undefined, so we didn't know yet its type or stage. He shared that what we wanted was for the estrogen and progesterone hormone receptor test results to come back as positive, as that meant it would be easier to treat long term, and that there was an additional test call HER2/neu that we would want to come back as negative as a positive result would indicate a more aggressive type of breast cancer.

He actually covered every single question I had before I even needed to ask them. All of this before ever examining me, which put me completely at ease. Then it was time to change clothes for the first breast exam. When he left the room, Weezer looked at me and said, "I wish he had been my surgeon. You don't need me here anymore. I can tell you've got this."

And she was right.

I felt comfortable with him and I was ready for whatever his next instructions were.

Dr. Breast Surgeon again assured me that my spot was quite small, and we agreed that with the small size, that the most logical approach would be a lumpectomy and five days of radiation.

However, with my positive family history of breast cancer, he recommended that I also get genetic testing done to see if I tested positive for the BRCA gene. A positive result would have us consider changing the course of surgery to a double mastectomy and possibly a hysterectomy, given the high rate of ovarian cancer or recurrence of breast cancer in BRCA positive individuals. His office would schedule an appointment for me to see Dr. Geneticist, the first of a long list of new players on my growing team.

He also suggested that we go ahead and move forward with me seeing a radiation oncologist, so that we were all prepared when the results of the pathology and the BRCA testing came back. I had a pitcher who had thrown me a curveball, a good catcher in Dr. Breast Surgeon, and I figured this would be my first-base person in this game of drafting my own team.

Lastly, just to make sure there wasn't anything we were missing, he suggested I have an MRI on both breasts. With my dense breast tissue, he wanted to make sure there wasn't anything hiding out, even though he assured me my mammogram only indicated that one small spot, and no one had felt any lumps.

I walked out of Dr. Breast Surgeon's office feeling lighter than air, relieved, and already in love with him and his kind bedside manner. After the horror stories I had heard, I was feeling pretty damn good. He had removed any fear I had and assured me that this was just a small spot, so it would be easy to treat.

The "Lucky Lows" strike again!

Radiation Treatment

Radiation therapy is a cancer treatment that uses high doses of radiation to kill cancer cells and to stop them from spreading.

More than 60 percent of people with cancer receive radiation therapy. For a fortunate number of lucky individuals, radiation is the *only* kind of cancer treatment they will require.

Radiation therapy can be an external beam (where the machine outside your body aims radiation at the cancer cells) or internal (where the radiation is put inside your body, near or in the cell or tumor).

Sometimes people get one kind or the other, and sometimes a few people get both kinds of radiation therapy.

Radiation may be given before, during, or after surgery. Your doctor may want to use radiation to shrink the size of a tumor before surgery, or they may want to use it to kill any remaining cells around the tumor site after surgery.

Radiation may also be given before, during, or after chemotherapy. Radiation therapy can shrink the tumor so that the chemotherapy works better. Sometimes, chemotherapy is given to help radiation therapy work better.

There are several people that may be involved in your radiation treatments. You will definitely see the radiation oncologist, and you may see any number of the rest of these teammates, depending on where you are receiving your therapy and who they have as support staff:

- **Radiation Oncologist:**
  This is a specially trained doctor who uses radiation therapy to treat cancer. They decide how much radiation you will receive, how your treatment will be given, follow you during your treatment, and prescribe any medication you should need if you experience any side effects.

- **Nurse Practitioner:**
  This is a nurse with advanced training who may take your medical history, do physical exams, order tests, manage side effects and watch your response to the treatment. They may even see you for some of your follow-up exams rather than the oncologist.

- **Radiation Nurse:**
  This person will provide nursing care, should you need it during your treatment, will talk with you about your treatment, and will work closely with the rest of your team to manage any side effects.

- **Radiation Therapist:**
  This person works with you during each radiation session. They will position you for the treatment and run the machines to make sure you get the dose of radiation prescribed for you by your radiation oncologist.

How you select your radiation oncologist is just like interviewing any of your other physicians. Prior to any appointments or having any treatments, you will want to make sure that they are CONTRACTED with your insurance company. If their practice is separate from the facility where they do the radiation, you will want to make sure the facility is CONTRACTED as well.

You will want to have a good relationship with this person as they may be the first, and if you are lucky, maybe the only physician who treats your cancer. When you meet them, you want to make sure that you get all of your questions answered before you leave their office.

Here are some questions that you may want to ask:

- What is my diagnosis?
- What Stage is my cancer?
- What are my treatment options? What are the benefits of each option? What are the side effects?
- Should I undergo genetic testing?
- Will I need any additional testing?
- What is the test for?
- What will the results of the additional testing tell you?
- When will you get the results? How will I be informed?
- Why do I need radiation?
- What is the goal of radiation?
- What are the benefits?
- What are the chances it will work?
- How often is this performed for my type of cancer?
- How many times have you done this for my type of cancer?
- What is your success rate?
- What are the possible complications, risks, or side effects?
- Why do I need this treatment?
- Do I have cancer in my lymph nodes?
- What is the significance of cancer found in the lymph nodes?

- Are there any other alternatives to treat the cancer?
- Will I need other cancer treatments, like chemotherapy or surgery, before or after radiation?
- What will happen if I don't have radiation?
- What do I have to lose or gain if I don't have radiation?
- Am I healthy enough to have radiation?
- Are you certified by a Specialty Radiation Board?
- Exactly what will be happening during radiation?
- Will the radiation cure the cancer?
- How long will the radiation take?
- Can I drive?
- Will I have to stay in the hospital? If so, how long?
- What happens if the radiation doesn't work?
- What can I expect after radiation? Will there be a lot of pain? Will I have any drains or catheters coming out of my body?
- Will I have an exit site that also needs to be treated?
- Can I sleep on my back, side, or stomach?
- How soon can I shower after radiation?
- Do I have any restrictions and if so, what are they and for how long?
- How will my body be affected by the radiation? Will it look or work differently? Will any of the changes be permanent?
- Will I be taking medicines after radiation? How do you spell it? How will I take it?
- Are there any side effects?
- Will this medicine be okay to take with my other medications?
- How soon can I go back to work?
- Do I need to change my daily routine?
- How long before I can go back to my usual activities like the gym?
- What about sex?
- Do you do the radiation here or somewhere else? If somewhere else, are they CONTRACTED with my insurance.

- Do I have time to get a second opinion?
- How quickly must I decide about my treatment?
- Will a delay in treatment reduce my chance of being cured?
- What is the percentage of developing a secondary cancer due to the radiation treatment?
- If I choose surveillance (monitoring of the cancer), or the cancer comes back, how will I be treated?
- What number should I call in an emergency?
- What is the name of the person I should communicate with in your office? Do they have a direct number?

These last two questions are usually addressed with the person responsible for billing:

- Will my insurance pay for this treatment?
- How much will my portion be?

You should never leave the radiologist's appointment with unanswered questions, unless they are about tests or pathology results that have not yet been completed.

EXTERNAL RADIATION:

At the time of this writing, radiation is usually either external or internal radiation although, depending on when you read this, there are innovators working on promising new therapies that by the time you hold this book, might be an option for your type of cancer. Be sure to ask if there are any new types of radiotherapy available for your type of cancer.

Prior to starting your radiation therapy, you will have a one-to two-hour meeting with your radiation oncologist and maybe even additional members of your radiation team. At this time, you will have a physical exam, your medical history will be reviewed, and you may have additional imaging.

At that appointment or on another day, depending on how soon your treatment will start, your radiation oncologist and therapist will define your treatment area or field. This is the area on your body that will get radiation. You will be scanned and/or x-rayed. During this you will be asked to lie very still while the therapist runs the tests to define the treatment area. Once the area has been defined, the radiation therapist will put small marks on your skin to specify the treatment area. Sometimes these marks are just temporary and will be left there only for the duration of your treatment; sometimes more permanent marks are put on your skin. These permanent marks are about the size of a small mole or freckle and are usually tattooed on your skin in order for the therapist to accurately position you for each treatment.

Depending on the location of your cancer, you may require a body mold that will help keep you from moving during each treatment. This mold is usually plastic foam, plastic, or plaster that will be shaped around your body to hold you comfortably in perfect position.

If you are receiving radiation to the head, you may need a mask. Although it sounds frightening, it is more like a plastic mesh that has air holes, and holes that will be cut for your eyes, nose and mouth. This mesh mask covers your head and attaches to the table while you receive your treatments. This keeps your head from moving and holds you in the exact same position for each of your treatments.

Once you have been marked and molded, you will be given a schedule of your appointments. Some doctors like to do a practice run the day before they start actual treatment, so you become comfortable with the entire process and you can get any last-minute questions answered.

On the days of your appointments, wear comfortable clothing. You may be asked to change into a robe or hospital gown depending on what area of the body you are receiving radiation. Once in your gown, you will be taken into a waiting room and then the treatment room where you will receive your radiation.

Depending on where your cancer is located, you will either sit in a chair or lie down on a special treatment table. The therapist will use colored lights on your skin to position you for treatment each day. These are only for positioning. Once you are positioned, the radiation therapist will leave the room. They are in a nearby room to control the radiation machine. They also watch you through a window or on a TV screen, so you are really never alone.

During the treatment, you cannot, hear, see, feel, or smell the radiation. Radiation therapy does not hurt while it is being given.

Your entire visit may last from 30 minutes to an hour. The reality is that most of this time is spent getting you aligned in the correct position. Most radiation treatments last about one to five minutes.

There may be times during your treatment that your radiation oncologist will want you to have a scan or an X-ray. This is not unusual and should not concern you that anything is wrong. The purpose is to make sure you are being positioned accurately during your treatments. This should add a measure of comfort to know they are keeping a close eye on you.

INTERNAL RADIATION:

Internal Radiation (also called brachytherapy) differs in that instead of the radiation coming from a machine on the outside of your body, the radiation is placed inside your body in the form of seeds, ribbons, or capsules that are placed in or near the cancer cells. This allows treatment with a higher dose of radiation to a smaller portion of your body. Internal radiation can also be in liquid form (that you receive by drinking), in the form of a pill, or through an IV. Liquid radiation travels through your body hunting for the cancer cells and killing them.

Just like external radiation, prior to starting your internal radiation therapy, you will have a one to two-hour meeting with your radiation oncologist and maybe even additional members of your radiation team. At this time, you will have a physical exam, your medical history will be reviewed, and you may have additional imaging. Your doctor will review the type of radiation they think is best for you, its benefits, and side effects and will instruct you on how to care for yourself during and after treatment.

For brachytherapy, the seeds, ribbons, or capsules are put in place through a small stretchy tube called a catheter or a larger device called an applicator. Your doctor will place the catheter or applicator into the part of your body being treated.

You will most likely be in the hospital when your catheter or applicator is put in place. This is what you can expect:

- You will be put to sleep, or the area where the catheter goes will be numbed.
- The catheter or applicator will be placed in your body by your doctor.
- If you are just numbed, you will be asked to lie very still while the insertion takes place. If you feel any discomfort, tell the doctor or nurse, and they can use more numbing medication to make you comfortable.

Once the treatment plan has been decided upon and the catheter or applicator has been put in place, the radiation source may be kept in place for a few minutes, days, or even the rest of your life. How long the radiation is in place depends on the type of cancer you have, where it is in your body, your health, and any other cancer treatments you have had or might need. Your radiation oncologist will discuss this with you.

Once the radiation source is in place, your body will give off radiation. With brachytherapy, your bodily fluids will not give off radiation; however, with liquid radiation, your body fluids will give off radiation for a while. Your doctor or nurse will talk with you about any safety measures you will need to take.

Sometimes brachytherapy is given in very high dosages. Some safety measures may include:

- Hospitalization in a private room to protect others and quick treatment by your nurse and other hospital staff. They will always provide the care you need, but they may stand or talk with you from a distance.
- Visitors may not be allowed.
- If you are allowed visitors, they will need to check in with the hospital staff before they enter your room.
- Visits may be kept short.
- Children and pregnant women are usually not allowed to visit.
- You may need to take certain precautions or follow some safety measures once you are no longer in the hospital, but your doctor or nurse will cover that in detail prior to your release.

When they remove the catheter or applicator, you might get medication for pain and you may find that the area where it was located may be tender for a few months. But once the catheter or applicator is removed, there is no longer radiation in your body. You also may find that you need to limit strenuous activities for a week or two, but always follow the instructions of your radiologist.

SIDE EFFECTS:

The most common side effects from radiation are skin changes and fatigue. Otherwise, most people find that they can generally go about their daily business and routine without much difficulty.

The skin changes often feel like a sunburn and can include dryness, itching, peeling, or even blistering. You will need to take extra special care of your skin during radiation. If the changes are serious, make sure to report them to your doctor as there are prescription medications that can help with these side effects.

Fatigue during radiation is quite common and there is a good chance you will feel some level of fatigue at some point in your treatment, or even a few weeks after your treatment is completed. You can manage some of this by:

- Making sure you get at least 8 hours of sleep each night.
- Exercising, because even just a brisk 10-minute walk can decrease the fatigue symptoms significantly. Do more if you can but be sure to first check with your radiologist about any exercise regimen outside of walking.
- Schedule a rest time. You may find you cannot get through the day without an afternoon nap. Many people find it helpful to take a short 10- to 15-minute rest. If you do nap, try not to sleep for more than an hour at a time as it may make it more difficult to sleep at night.

If you are having radiation to your head or neck, you may be instructed to visit your dentist at least two weeks before your treatment starts. This is so your dentist can examine your teeth and mouth to make sure your mouth is as healthy as possible before therapy begins. If you cannot get to the dentist before your treatment starts, tell your radiologist and ask for their guidance.

There can be other side effects depending on the part of your body being treated. These can include diarrhea, hair loss, mouth changes, nausea or vomiting, throat changes, urinary and bladder changes, shortness of breath, cough, earaches, taste changes, headaches, blurry vision, and sexual and fertility changes. You should tell your doctor if you are experiencing any of these changes as there are suggested ways that many of these side effects, if not all, can be managed.

Once you have finished radiation therapy, you will need follow-up care for the rest of your life. This specific follow-up care refers to checkups with your radiation oncologist or nurse practitioner after your radiation is completed. During these checkups, your doctor or nurse will check to see how well the radiation therapy worked, check for other signs of cancer, check for any late side effects, or order lab and imaging tests. These may include blood tests, X-rays, CT, MRI or PET scans. These appointments get further apart the longer you are cancer-free.

• • •

Tips:

- Take your three-ring binder.
- Take someone with you and/or record the visit.
- Make a copy of the above questions to take with you. (You can download a copy at www.holycrapihavecancer.com .) Cross out, ahead of time, all the questions you already know the answer to, or that are not pertinent to you or your type of cancer, so that you can skip right over those.
- Make your notes on the question sheet you have copied.
- Do not leave your first appointment without getting all your questions answered.

- Follow your gut!
- Transfer the answers to the notes section in your three-ring binder.
- It is best that you not begin asking questions until your doctor is finished explaining what they know and then asks if you have any questions. Most doctors cover most of these questions as they explain your situation. If, at the end, they don't ask if you have questions, when it seems like they have covered everything, let them know you have a few questions. Keep this sheet handy and review each and every question, until you feel ALL of your questions have been answered.
- Remember that this is an interview with the person that now has your life in their hands. Treat it like that.
- Arrive on time for all your appointments.
- When being set up for your mold or mask, make sure you get positioned in the most comfortable way possible. When they create your mold or mask, this will be your position during all your radiation treatments. Do not be afraid to tell your technician you are not comfortable and work with them until you are satisfied.
- Tell your therapist or doctor if you are having any pain.
- Follow the instructions of your radiation team about taking care of your skin, drinking liquids, and eating the foods on your diet.
- Immediately tell your doctor if you are having any changes to your skin.
- Some people do not want to have the permanent tattoos put on their body to be utilized for treatment placement. If you are one of these individuals, you will need to let the radiation oncologist know at the initial visit. There are ways to get around these permanent marks, but they require additional work by

the therapy team and may require for longer appointment times for your treatment, so make sure you communicate this desire in advance, so they can accommodate your request.

- Be sure to tell the radiation therapist if you feel sick or uncomfortable. They can stop the machine at any time.
- Bring something to read, or whatever can occupy your time, in the waiting room.
- Plan your therapy schedule at a time that makes sense for you. For example, you might want to have your treatment on your way to work, over a lunch hour, or at the end of the day on your way home.
- Exercise *really does* make a difference.
- Notify your doctor immediately if you have any dramatic changes.
- If your radiation is in your rectal area, use baby wipes or a spray bottle to cleanse yourself. Also, ask your doctor or nurse about sitz baths, which are warm water baths taken in a sitting position with just enough water to cover the affected area.
- If your rectal area becomes sore, tell your doctor.
- Regardless of your sex, prior to treatment let your doctor know if you are wanting to have children. They will cover ways to preserve your fertility before treatment starts.
- Discuss any sexual or fertility changes with your doctor.
- For mouth pain: sip water often during the day. Suck on ice chips. Chew sugar-free gum or suck on sugar-free candy. Keep your mouth clean. Use an extra soft toothbrush. Do not use mouthwash that contains alcohol. If these things do not help, consult your doctor.

- Use only products on your skin that your doctor or nurse suggests or agrees are acceptable to use.
- Wear clothes that are not tight and can breathe. Avoid pantyhose and form fitting clothes.
- Avoid extreme temperatures on your skin such as ice packs or heating pads. That means showering or bathing with lukewarm water.
- Communicate any urinary or bladder changes to your doctor.
- Drink plenty of fluids.

• • •

Ann's Tips:

All my doctors were amazed at how great my skin remained throughout my radiation treatment and post therapy as well. To this day they all comment on it when I go to get fondled, uh, I mean, examined for follow-up appointments. Here's the process I utilized and what you will need, but always confirm its use with your team prior to starting and know that by the time you are reading this, there may have been other skin sparing treatments created:

- Pure Lanolin. (I liked one from *now solutions* that I purchased on Amazon. I preferred this brand as it had the consistency of petroleum jelly and would stay on my skin much longer. If you are allergic to lanolin just use the Aquaphor.)
- *Aquaphor Advanced Therapy Healing Ointment.* (This can be found at most drugstores and online.)
- Old t-shirts. (Depending on where you are having radiation you might want sweatpants, cotton underwear, or a soft scarf or make a scarf from a strip of flannel. Just

make sure it is something you do not care about as it is going to become oily and greasy.)

- Cheap Sports Bra. (If you're having radiation to your breasts.)
- Sheets you do not care about.

Instructions:

o Before going to bed, slather the lanolin all over the affected area of your body. Put on the t-shirt or sweatpants, or wrap the soft scarf or strip of flannel in place. Sleep with the lanolin on the affected area all night.

o You will be instructed to make sure that area is clean of any lotions or medicine prior to radiation so you will need to adjust the rest of this *Tip* around your radiation and work schedule. I'm lucky to have a home office, so I was able to apply it all day. Just know there is no wrong way to do it. The idea is to keep that area as soft and moisturized as possible, for as long as possible, during the treatment.

o If I didn't have to leave my home office in the morning, I slathered more on, put on a sports bra, and went for a walk. My radiation was mid-morning, so I went to my radiation appointment right after showering to remove ALL the ointment. (Make sure you soap that area well to remove any residual ointment.)

o After radiation, if I wasn't going anywhere, I slathered more lanolin all over the area and put on the yucky t-shirt. If I had to go anywhere, I used the Aquaphor, with a cheap bra, so I didn't smell like a wet sheep. (Know that both the lanolin and the Aquaphor may bleed through your clothing, so prepare accordingly. That is also the reason for the sheets you don't care about. Even with clothing or a scarf to cover it, it may

bleed through your clothing and ruin your sheets. I just used things I knew I was going to throw out when I was done.)
- o Re-apply lanolin at bedtime. Sleep, slather, repeat.

My fatigue didn't hit until two weeks after my radiation was completed. Several of my cancer brothers and sisters recommended many things, but this are the one thing I think that helped the most.

- **Exercise.** It really did make a difference. I walked at least 10 minutes every day, longer when treatment and work allowed me. If you are being treated with chemo or having any type of surgery during your radiation treatments, you will want to first okay this with those doctors before starting.

• • •

My Story:

Two days after my appointment with Dr. Breast Surgeon, I met with Dr. Geneticist for the BRCA testing, five days later I was scheduled for an MRI, and eight days later I had an appointment with Dr. Radiation Oncologist.

In my mind, everything was moving along smoothly to schedule the lumpectomy and radiation; unless, of course, the BRCA test came back as positive, which would change the course of what we would be doing.

However, I was already ready to be DONE and we hadn't even started.

Money was a HUGE concern for us. Well, more so for me, as I ALWAYS seem to worry about money. But having said that, in order to be able to afford the premiums for our affordable healthcare, we had to carry extremely high deductibles. I had told all the doctors I wanted to have everything completed by the end of the year, so we would only have to meet our deductible once. I didn't want to have to figure out how to come up with a large deductible, and then worry about how to do it all over again at the beginning of 2015, only 4 months away. So I was pleased with the speed with which everything was occurring.

On August 14, as I was leaving for my appointment to meet with Dr. Radiologist, I received an expected call from Dr. Breast Surgeon, but with results that weren't expected. He explained to me that the results of the MRI showed I had two more suspicious areas and it showed possible lymph node involvement, so I was no longer a candidate for a lumpectomy. He also said that the pathology results had come back with the estrogen and progesterone results positive, as we had hoped, but the HER2/neu had come back as positive, which meant I would need chemotherapy.

[WHAAAAAT??? You have got to be FREAKING kidding me? THAT was NOT part of the game plan!!! Remember? Lumpectomy? 5 days of radiation? Done by the end of the year? WHAT. THE. HELL!!!!]

He also suggested that I have the two suspicious spots biopsied so we were certain they were indeed malignant, not just pissed off from the previous biopsy. And we might as well have me see a plastic surgeon to at least have a conversation about reconstruction, so I would have that information to mull over.

Oh, yeah, and I would now need to meet Dr. Medical Oncologist to discuss chemotherapy. He suggested that I keep my appointment with Dr. Radiation Oncologist as I would

STILL need radiation at some point down the road and he would call Dr. Radiologist to give her an update.

[THIS! CANNOT! BE! HAPPENING!]

Talk about a game changer and we weren't even out of the first inning.

However, I continued to move forward by meeting with Dr. Radiation Oncologist.

And I immediately liked d her as she also had a calming demeanor and I could tell we would work well together.

She explained radiation and why I would need it. I could tell from her conversation that she was still looking at the original plan of a lumpectomy and five days of radiation. At that point I asked her if she had heard from Dr. Breast Surgeon, and she said she had received a message, but they were unable yet to speak in person. I shared with her, as best I could, what he had told me. Even being a rookie to the game, I was already starting to use the alphabet soup that I was quickly becoming familiar with. Now, instead of RBIs and ERAs, I was tossing out terms like MRIs, BRCA, and HER2/neu. Apparently, cancer was going to lend itself to the easy record-keeping and statistics, just like baseball.

Dr. Radiologist listened to me. She then said that it was quite possible that the additional suspicious areas could just be inflamed from the previous biopsy and they might be nothing at all. She also shared her opinion that the MRI results could be an over interpretation, especially given there were no signs of the tumors during all my breast exams or on my mammogram. She thought that I should just proceed with the MRI biopsy and BRCA testing and that she would connect with Dr. Breast Surgeon and get clarity. But she assured me I would see her again, as I would still require radiation; now we just weren't sure when.

Waiting (You've Been Benched!)

No player wants to sit on the bench or straighten bats and helmets while waiting your turn to get into the game.

Unfortunately, there is A LOT of bench warming in cancer.

LOTS of waiting.

Waiting for calls.

And for appointments.

And results.

Staging.

Hospital calls.

Pathology reports.

Waiting. Waiting. Waiting.

Did I mention, there is an incredible amount of waiting involved when you are diagnosed with cancer?

Until I was diagnosed, I had no idea that getting all the information required to make the best decision sometimes takes a while.

How about FOREVER? Or that's the way it seems!

It is difficult enough to cope with a cancer diagnosis, but if you must wait a few weeks or more for important appointments, scans, or results before treatment can start, you might possibly — and rightfully so — become anxious, frightened, and frustrated. It's easy to be concerned that the cancer may be spreading while all this waiting is going on. Fortunately, cancers usually grow slowly, so this is not likely to happen.

There is always a chance that your cancer has spread to other parts of the body. Because of this, doctors do a variety of tests to confirm cancer location. These additional scans and tests are valuable so that you and your doctors have as much information as possible. This helps them stage your cancer; knowing the stage of your cancer helps your doctor determine which treatment strategy is best for you.

Unfortunately, those things DO take time. Waiting for the appointment. Waiting for the results. You may have to go to a special outpatient facility or hospital where their schedules might be booked full for a couple of weeks.

Waiting.

There also may be a waiting time while your doctors work to get the test or procedure prior authorized with your insurance. (Unless you have unlimited resources, never have any of these tests or procedures done without insurance pre-approval. Pushing ahead without prior authorization, regardless of how quickly you WANT to get your answers, may have you paying expenses out of pocket that could have been avoided if you had just been a bit more patient.)

I know. I know. I'm an instant gratification junkie myself; but patience must become a part of the journey.

Waiting!!

There is waiting, and you must be patient. I'm not saying you have to like it, but you will need to be patient. A three-minute egg still takes three minutes.

• • •

Tips:

- There will be waiting. Be prepared for that; especially at each new doctor appointment. If you need to, carry water and snacks (unless you've been told not to eat.)
- Self-care, even in the beginning, should be non-negotiable.
- Put these self-care activities as events on your calendar; that way you are reminded to do them. Your calendar will fill quickly in the next few weeks or months. If you truly make self-care non-negotiable, you want to make sure nothing interrupts these activities. Or if they are going to be interrupted, be sure that you can reschedule them. Putting them on your calendar — and actually treating them like appointments — makes self-care a daily habit.
- Communicate with whomever you live with that you have set aside these times and request to be left alone. You may find you have to go to another room and shut the door. Maybe even lock it. Whatever it takes, make it happen. I let Hubby know it was also for his well-being. I knew if I didn't keep my anxiety under control that he might one night be having a visit from Mr. Pillow while I got in a 5-minute cardio workout holding it over his face.
- Find whatever activity works for your anxiety and make whatever adjustments you need. I could not sit cross-

legged, so I would lie flat on my back with a pillow rolled up under my knees. I still do guided meditation this way.

- Move your body every day. In the beginning, I could do pretty much everything I always had. I walked. I hiked. I went to the gym. As chemotherapy progressed, that was less easy. I know it is 57 steps, one way, to my workshop and nine steps to the swing on my back patio. There were a few days that those steps were the extent of my moving, but I made sure I moved at least once every day. Maybe from bed to couch is all you can accomplish? Well, it's still moving.

- If none of these tools are helping with your anxiety, speak with your doctor. Some degree of anxiety, depression, and sleep changes are very common during this time. Do not be afraid to share it with one of your physicians. There is no reason to white knuckle this. It doesn't work. Speak up!

Ann's Tips:

Waiting, for me, was like a cruel punishment. As if being diagnosed with cancer wasn't enough, and now being told that it was probably a bit more than just a teeny weensy spot and five days of radiation, the little voice inside my head would not SHUT UP! I walked around like a little kid who had been admonished, "Wait until your father gets home!"

When I would wake up in the morning, there was always that brief few seconds when everything seemed right with the world. But after a second or two it was, "Oh yeah — I have cancer."

[NOOOOO!]

That little voice in my head was ALWAYS talking. And often it wasn't the most happy and upbeat of conversations. She was really great at "what if's" and catastrophizing. With a fresh brain, every morning that little voice immediately went in to overdrive with irrational thoughts.

Those first few days were excruciating, having all this minutia rattling around in my head.

[How are we going to pay for this? What should I do? Will I be sick? Who will take care of Mom? What about FIL AND MIL? I can't miss my daughter Landry's fashion show. What if I just don't do anything?]

I realized that, if I didn't find some releases for these negative mental gyrations, I was going to end up going down a very unproductive path.

I've spent a great deal of my adult life delving into personal development. Not so much because I think there is anything wrong with me, but because I want to be the best me possible. I also realized that it can be a mad, mad world out there and I wanted to be able to impart wisdom to my children that might make their worlds work better. Personal development is one of those things I am passionate about. I believe if we aren't learning something every day, we start dying. I choose personal development as one of those things I want to keep learning about.

But somehow with this thing called cancer, it was like EVERYTHING I had ever learned about keeping myself present, about not letting my stories in my head take over, and all the other tools I had used over the years to make my life run more smoothly just evaporated.

Poof. Gone. Inaccessible.

After receiving the news from Dr. Breast Surgeon that there might be more cancer there than originally detected, I realized I was so far out of my body and the unproductive conversations in my head were taking up every second that I was awake. I needed to do something about it. It's exhausting being in a tailspin before your first cup of coffee every day. Especially over something you have little or no control over: the appointments, the waiting, and the uncertainty. Reading the bad news in the newspaper would put me in a dark place. I could feel myself becoming more and more anxious. I felt out of control. I needed to go back to some of my training and find some simple things that would get me out of this hole. I still had our business to help run, Mom, MIL and FIL to care for and I still needed to get myself to doctor appointments.

I needed to get off the crazy train!

Standing in front of my library of personal development books, I just asked the universe to assist me in finding the best tools that would help get me through the next few months. I know, it's a little woo-woo and fairy dust-ish; but it's pretty amazing what the universe will provide, if you just ask. Over the years it has worked very well for me, so I figured I had nothing to lose.

It was while standing there that I had a flash of a memory of how much journaling had helped me in the past. I was a nearly daily journal writer for many years. But as life got busy, I hadn't done any journaling for quite some time. I realized that this might be a great time to revisit it. I needed to do something with all this worry that was bouncing around between my ears like a ball in a pinball machine. I was determined not to burden anyone else with something that tens of thousands of people before me had gone through. I'm not a pussy for Christ's sake! At the time, it seemed a bother to say the things that were in my head and I NEVER want to be a bother! I thought this just might be the ticket.

I immediately started what I would come to refer to as my **Morning Mind Puke**.

Morning Mind Pukes are three pages of HANDWRITTEN script of WHATEVER was in my head. The little worrying voice inside my head talked a mile a minute and had a lot of neurotic things to say. I figured if I got those things out of my head and onto paper, I might be able to feel like I was back in my body.

I decided I would try writing every day for a week. If it wasn't helping, I would quit and look for something else to help me disembark from the crazy train. I just knew I had so many things unsaid in my head, but I just didn't feel up to "burdening" anyone with what, at the time, were feelings that I thought were exclusive to me. (Oh, how wrong I was about THAT little selfish thought.) At this point we hadn't told anyone else, and I wasn't planning on telling anyone else. So how could I get rid of the garbage ricocheting inside my head when I wasn't ready to share it with anyone yet?

So, I began to write. Three pages. No more. No less. And I had rules that seemed to help:

- It had to be THE first thing I did every morning. I got up, drank 8 to 10 ounces of water (a good way to start any day), made coffee, and by the time it was done brewing, I would sit down to write. No reading the paper. No TV. No news. No going out to walk or to the gym until my three pages were done. No exceptions.

- These mind pukes were meant for me and me alone. No one else could read them except me. I didn't even re-read them. I would write them and, as a ritual, I would promptly shred them. And while I shredded them, I would say in my head, "Okay, I'm done with these thoughts for today." Yes, more woo-woo, but that ritual actually worked! And if those thoughts would resurface throughout the day, which they often would (the work of an obsessive brain), I would say to my little voice, "NOPE, you've already dealt with this today and released it. Let it go. If it comes back tomorrow deal with it then, but for now you are done with those thoughts." It sounds crazy, but it actually began to work from the very first day.

- There was no wrong way to do this. It didn't matter what was on those pages, I just needed to get it on paper. The pages weren't meant to sound smart or be some well-thought-out journal. It was merely the act of moving the hand across the page and writing WHATEVER came to mind. No structure. No detail or neatness. Since I was trying to retain my sanity in this ever-changing situation, there was nothing off limits. Afraid of the results of the BRCA — I wrote about it. What was this going to cost us — I wrote about it. Woke up feeling optimistic — I wrote about it. Mad that the cat puked on the carpet — I wrote about it. Nothing was off limits. Nothing too silly, too stupid, too insignificant, or too strange to include. One day I filled the three pages with nothing but, "I'm so tired of this shit!" Over and over and over again, until I filled three pages.

- Always three pages – no matter what.

For you, like me, a Morning Mind Puke might often be negative, stilted, full of self-pity, fragmented, repetitive, boring, childish, filled with anger — even filled with feelings you aren't even able to recognize. GREAT! WRITE THAT SHIT DOWN!!!!

All that stuff that is knocking around in your head is keeping you from being present in your situation and empowered on the journey. Whatever you are worrying about — work, insurance, who will watch the kids while I'm in the hospital, who will drive me, why is Hubby being such a dick — whatever stuff muddies your thoughts — GET IT ON PAPER! Then let it go!

Meditation: Medication for the Brain

I also realized I needed to work on breathing. I was so amped up most of the time that I would be going along and realize I wasn't really breathing.

[How would I get in my appointment in the morning and the two afternoon doctor appointments for Mom and FIL? Why hadn't I heard back on the BRCA testing? When will I hear from Dr. Breast Surgeon with what's next? Why hasn't my insurance called?]

I would find myself literally holding my breath and having to remind myself to breathe.

I have many friends for which meditation is a daily practice and they swear by it. I struggled for years with meditation as I pictured people sitting cross-legged OM'ing their way to peace. First, for me, sitting cross-legged on the floor was uncomfortable. It hurts my hips. I hated it. Second, all the OM'ing on the planet would not shut up the little voice in my head.

[This is stupid. Did you eat breakfast? Are we done yet? My back hurts? Shit, forgot to pay the liability insurance.]

I convinced myself that I'm just one of those people who CAN'T meditate.

Then one day, a few years prior to all of this, I read an interesting article about meditation that made plenty of sense to me. This author felt that anything you do with rhythmic movement could be considered meditation. THAT worked for me. I love riding my bicycle and I recall feeling the most at peace when I was into the rhythm of my pedaling. Walking worked the same way for me. Moving my body and REALLY paying attention to what muscles I was using, or the rhythm of my steps made me feel more grounded, calmer.

After the first biopsy, I was quite sore, so going to the gym was not always an option. Walking became my daily moving meditation. A walking meditation. One foot in front of the other. But I needed to have music going or the little voice in my head would be jabbering away.

But by most afternoons I was again feeling pretty anxious. I decided to dig out some of my old guided meditations I had purchased years ago. You know — all those CDs still in their shrink wrap. I went through my library and didn't find anything that appealed to me when that little voice reminded me that this was no longer 1990 and they have things called smartphones. Wouldn't you know there was a dizzying array of apps to choose from? Duh!

I overwhelm easily with too many choices, so my modus operandi is, when overwhelmed, to do nothing. Not really a winning strategy. So, I went to a trusted source for important information . . . Facebook. Within minutes of posting the question: "What meditation apps do you like?" I had several suggestions that I narrowed down to two that seemed to suit me: OMG I Can Meditate (now called Breethe: Sleep and Meditation) and Headspace. Over time OMG became my favorite as there were time-based meditations — some as short as two minutes — and others to choose from as well. Later, I used one that I found particularly useful, Chemotherapy Meditation.

Now I had three things to do daily that helped me feel like I was a little bit more in control of the stuff going on inside my head.

Morning Mind Puke, **Moving Meditation,** and **Guided Meditation**. I used them daily and recommend them to you as well. Although going crazy is certainly an option, (and I have met some on the cancer journey that have chosen this route) now is really a good time to try to stay as present and as in control as possible.

In the beginning, I found the waiting the most challenging part. Having tools to lessen that frustration helped me and can assist you through this process and perhaps decrease some of the anxiety often attributed to a cancer diagnosis.

• • •

My Story:

At this point we were waiting for the BRCA results, which were supposed to take about seven to ten days. These results were going to determine possible surgical options.

I had been told by Dr. Geneticist that if there were any issues with my insurance I would be contacted by the lab; if there were no challenges, they would proceed with the test without calling me. I never received a call so assuming there were no issues, we waited.

And waited.

And waited.

After 10 days with no word, I was getting concerned that I hadn't heard anything. I contacted the lab where the testing was being done to see if I could find out where in the process my results were. When I was finally able to speak with someone who could, after much delay and searching, locate my file and specimen, they explained that my lab work had not been processed yet because my insurance was not going to cover the test. Someone was supposed to have called me to let me know this, as their policy is to not proceed with the test, if your insurance won't pay for it, without verbal communication and then signed documents from the patient agreeing to pay for the test out of pocket. She wasn't sure why no one had contacted me, but my sample had lingered on someone's desk for a week.

[WHAAAAT! THE! HELL!]

How was that possible? I was furious, deflated, and pretty much a crazy woman after that conversation. Didn't they realize that my treatment plan was going to be determined by the outcome of this test? And now we had just wasted 10 days.

[DAMMIT!]

I promptly called Dr. Breast Surgeon to let him know what I had discovered. His office reassured me that I was fine, we were okay to wait for the results, AND they would call Dr. Geneticist's office to request that the lab move my sample to the front of the line and rush the results.

Suddenly $4000 poorer, I was in a tailspin.

Deep breath!

Another deep breath.

I was quickly becoming a basket case.

Fortunately, I was also busy taking Mom and FIL to doctor appointments. A busy basket case. Between Mom, FIL, and myself, I went to or took someone to 18 doctor appointments *between the day I was diagnosed on August 4 to September 5. 18 doctor appointments, scans or tests in 20 days. I was beginning to feel like Gumby, stretched one way and then another. During the night, I would return to original shape only to be tugged and pulled different directions all over again the next day. It was a very chaotic time and I still didn't feel like we had any definitive plan.*

Waiting.

Who/How to Tell

Deciding **WHO** and **HOW** to tell people about your cancer is a very private decision. And it isn't necessarily an easy decision to make. In my hundreds of conversations with other cancer patients and survivors, I have heard probably every version possible of who they told, how, and their reasoning behind it. Tell no one. Tell just a few people. Tell your kids/don't tell your kids. To tell or not tell your family. Set up a website. Or every day update, share symptoms, setbacks, conversations, and pictures loud and proud on Facebook or Instagram.

This is a decision **YOU** will need to make for yourself.

You may be an introvert; you may be an extrovert. You may love your brother, but haven't spoken to your sister in 20 years. You may be someone that shares every little detail of your life with everyone, or you may be a very private person. You may be out in public a lot; you may never have to leave the house. You may have just a few close friends; you may have a million.

Whoever you are, **YOU** get to choose **WHO** and **HOW** to tell.

And it may not be easy.

It wasn't for me. I talk a lot, once you get me going, yet I'm pretty much a very private person. I've mastered the art of superficial conversation. With the original diagnosis of a small spot and five days of radiation, I hadn't planned to tell anyone. I've had worse things happen to me that I hadn't ever told anyone; so, I felt no need to share this.

However, we did decide to tell the kids. Intellectually, I knew that they now had an immediate family history of cancer that they would need to convey when they saw their physicians in the future and it was something that should be in their medical records. Emotionally, because we are a very close family, I knew they would be **PISSED** not to know. But in my heart, I didn't want to tell **anyone**.

My first exposure to the thought that I WOULD **have** to share my diagnosis with more than just the ones that already knew — our kids, Mom, MIL and FIL, and Weezer — came at the hands of Dr. Geneticist.

After documenting my family tree and reviewing our family health history, Dr. Geneticist told me that, if my BRCA test came back positive, I would need to have my children tested. She also told me that I would need to tell my surviving sibling, my brother. I told her that I had not told my brother, nor did I have any intention of telling him, that I had cancer. I don't like attention. I don't like sympathy. I had no intention of telling anyone else!

I remember the "Telephone Game" from elementary school; you sit in a circle; a person starts by whispering something into the ear of the person sitting next to them and by the time it gets all the way around the circle, what was originally said is nothing like what the last person repeats. Much is lost in the repetition from one person to the next. I knew that would be the case if I told just one person. So . . .I wasn't going to tell anyone. I didn't want it to go from no big deal to someone thinking I was about to be planted in the ground. Soblem prolved, as my daughter says.

Shocked might be the best description for Dr. Geneticist's facial expression when I told her I had no intention of telling my remaining sibling. She told me that I could do whatever I wanted; I was under no requirement to tell anyone. But, if I had any kind of conscience at all, with my positive family history and now my own diagnosis, I really had an obligation to at least tell my brother. Her very strong opinion was that he had a right to know so that he and his children would have this information to add to *their* medical history.

Oh, the words that little voice in my head was spewing! She was not happy!

Getting in my car, after the appointment, I remember immediately calling Hubby to vent to him about what she had said. I was selfishly unhappy — seething is probably more accurate — that I was now being forced into a position to have to tell someone outside of those who already knew.

[Great! Another thing out of my control!]

Over dinner I whined to my husband about this strong opinion of Dr. Geneticist about my need to share the news with others. I was still unhappy about it.

Then I started thinking about all the people I love: Mama Bear, The Chef, Cowboy, Little League Husband (the person I work closely with running Little League), Foot Massager, The Visitor, The Cowgirl...the list goes on and on, and I realized I would be *PISSED* if they were going through something like this and didn't tell me. FURIOUS!!

With that in mind, I stayed up after Hubby went to bed and did what seems to always work best for me — I put it to paper. I wrote. What would I say to the people that I thought would want to know? I just wrote away and decided to sleep on it.

The next morning, I had pretty much decided to just let my very closest of friends know. Then I realized another good friend knew one of those close friends, so the list grew. I'm blessed to have friends all over the world, and I knew a few of them would want to know as well. The list continued to grow. I was actually becoming nauseated as the list grew. I became even more queasy as the list grew even longer.

But even worse, I got more and more woozy as I thought about people just knowing at all.

I HATE confrontation and will do just about anything to avoid it. This felt even worse. Way worse!

Why, you ask?

Telling people finally made it seem real.

I now knew, in my heart, that if I told anyone, there was not going to be an eventual call from Dr. Vaginacologist telling me this was all some big mistake.

I wasn't going to wake up and it was some scary dream.

There would be no turning back.

For the first time, I was faced with knowing — *like NO SHIT* — I really had cancer.

This was the worst I had felt since hearing, "I'm sorry, but you have cancer." In that moment, I realized that by telling others, it was finally real. It wasn't going to go away.

But something surprising happened as well. For the first time, I felt like I wasn't on the outside looking in. Suddenly, I was back in my body.

That made me realize something else. Suddenly, I was ready to face what was ahead. Like no kidding READY!

[Bring it on!]

Yippee! I had my **who** would be told.

Now, I had to figure out **how** to tell them.

I certainly knew I wasn't going to call everyone. I actually HATE talking on the telephone, especially the cell phone. Too much background noise, the phone breaks up, I'm either too loud or not loud enough.

I also have a terrible time verbally recreating conversations. I leave out stuff. I get the order of things all wrong. I make the story more confusing. So, that was not an option.

I could email everyone, but I didn't have everyone's email. Also, it was 2014 and more people were communicating via text and less by email. And I definitely didn't have everyone's cell numbers to text.

But nearly everyone I thought would want to know WAS on Facebook. Yup, I did the thing I **NEVER** thought I would do; I went to Mark Zuckerberg's invention to let my friends and family know I had cancer.

[Are you kidding me? Do you have any idea how tacky that is? Do you have no couth?]

Despite the little voice's non-stop abusive discourse about the inappropriateness of sharing something this important in this manner, I decided to create a group message to those that were on Facebook and the few not on Facebook I would email.

After taking a walk, drinking multiple cups of coffee, and rereading and editing what I had written what felt like 100 times, with shaking hand, my right index finger hovered over the send button until I finally had the courage and pushed send with this message:

I'll start with an apology.

First for the length of this message and second, because I know this is not the best way to share important news. But you all know me pretty well and know I despise talking on the telephone; and this is really the most efficient way to share my new adventure — which currently has me a little busy.

So, if you are getting this message, you are important to me! AND I thought you might want to know what's the haps. This way the next time we see each other I don't have to vomit this minutia all over you should you ask what I've been up to, and I can just brag about my kids and complain about gas prices instead.

You know – the usual.

For sake of efficiency I will get right to the point . . . I have been diagnosed with breast cancer. Don't even go to OMG that's awful, horrible, tragic news or any of those thoughts. It's not. First, because I say so. Second, because it has been found very early so that gives us lots of options. It was discovered early enough that the site is about the size of the head of a big nail. Which, given the size of my breasticles, makes it almost microscopic.

So, here's the scoop: the next few weeks are going to be a whirlwind of activity. I've already met my new best friend (Dr. Breast Surgeon) and we have discussed the options.

First, I will have additional testing (Dr. MRI) to make sure the girls aren't hiding anything we haven't already seen. Not likely, but what the heck – might as well make sure. Then I am going to have a BRCA test (Dr. Geneticist) to make sure that I don't have some mutated gene that would have additional breast cancer or ovarian cancer show up later. There is no reason to think it will come back positive, but if it does it changes our course of treatment. Since I'm determined to do this only once, it's important information to have. If all those things are fine, in about 3 to 4 weeks I will have a lumpectomy, have my lymph nodes poked, prodded and maybe removed and have 5 days of twice a day radiation (Dr. Radiation Oncologist). If the lymph nodes are clean (again no reason to think they aren't) then all is well and I will soon after meet another new friend (Dr. Medical Oncologist). He will prescribe the medication I will take for the rest of my life to ward off a recurrence (see above reference to only doing this once!).

I will see my new best friend (Dr. Breast Surgeon) very frequently – probably more often than I see many of you – for the next year and celebrate each passing year by getting to see him less frequently.

If the BRCA comes back positive I will have the breasticles lopped off and my ovaries removed which is a completely different ball game, and a longer recovery. But again, there is no reason to think that is the case – but always nice to know you have options.
So, if your reaction is "Holy Crap, Karma finally caught up with her!" you may be right.

If your reaction is "Damn, is there anything I can do?" Nope – not right now. The Lows are all great . . . yup, even me.

Just know that what's so is I have breast cancer, but it's early enough and we are going to be aggressive enough that I'm more likely to drop dead from old age than this.

If you want to connect with me – things haven't changed – text me. If you aren't Dr. Breast Surgeon, Dr. MRI, Dr. Geneticist, Dr. Radiation Oncologist or Dr. Medical Oncologist, I still more than likely won't answer the phone if you call. If you want to respond to this, please do so separately so everyone else isn't bothered with the blah, blah, blah.

And be certain of this – if you got this message – I pretty much love you!
Ann

Weeks later I sent this one:

New update – today the MRI came back showing two additional suspicious areas and possible lymph node involvement. My surgeon would like to do an MRI biopsy to find out if they are actually cancerous spots or not. But we have decided to wait the results of the BRCA and the MRI biopsy before any further decisions. If the MRI shows additional cancer the possibility of a lumpectomy is no longer an option and we would just proceed aggressively with the mastectomies. I'm telling you – these girls keep getting me in trouble! ☺

• • •

One of the things my friend and cancer mentor Terry coached me on was to not be surprised by the reactions of people once they heard the news. When I asked her what she meant by that, she said that regardless of how I decided to tell people, I wasn't going to make everyone happy. She shared that there would be people who would be unhappy that I hadn't called them directly or told them privately. She also warned me to be prepared for people saying incredibly insensitive things like "my mom just died from your kind of cancer."

She was right!

Fortunately, she had prepared me by sharing that if I received any kind of negative response, it was ALL about the other person and those people rarely stick around for the long haul. Again, she was correct.

Negative responses and insensitive things said have nothing to do with you. If someone calls you out on it, you do with it what you choose. Once you heard the word cancer, this became YOUR journey and you get to choose who, how, when, and even if you want to tell anyone.

If you are taking a traditional western medicine approach to treatment, telling people is one of the **FEW** things you have control over. Don't let anyone get in your head that you should have done it differently.

The other thing Terry shared was to be prepared to be surprised by who **REALLY** shows up, and to not be disappointed by those who don't. Every cancer patient I've talked to says this same thing. And it was so true for me. Through the entire process I was constantly so amazed and appreciative of those who hung in for the long haul. And mildly astonished by the ones who didn't, people I considered good friends who never once reached out. There is a quote I read somewhere: "You may never know who your true friends are until life throws you a curveball." No truer words were written.

Having cancer reminded me of when I was pregnant and not yet showing. I felt like I was walking around with a secret, yet I also felt like everyone should be able to tell that something was different. And like being pregnant, in the beginning, everyone wants to hear all about it, share their delivery horror stories, wish you well; but by about week 30 everyone is hoping for an early delivery — not too early, mind you — but early enough so you will stop obsessing about it. I wasn't really publicly talking about it all that much, but it certainly consumed every waking thought and many dinner table conversations.

Cancer can kind of drag on. You'll get fewer texts. Fewer people check on you. Your support team gets smaller. You'll probably find that just a handful will actually still be there to meet you at home plate when you hit the winning home run. That's just the nature of a long-drawn-out game. True fans stay until the last swing, and fair-weather fans hear about the walk-off home run on the radio in their car on their way home.

However, unexpectedly, several gifts came from telling people I had cancer. I knew — like **NO** kidding — who my real friends were. I had people that — like **NO** kidding — really cared about me and until I shared my situation, I had no idea the impact I had had on them. I learned — like **NO** kidding — who I would take a bullet for. If they stuck around for the long haul, I would slide down a banister of razor blades, into a pool of rubbing alcohol, and roll in salt for them.

I think as we age, we all get this lesson in friendship over time. But I think when you have cancer (or perhaps any critical illness), this occurs with velocity.

• • •

Tips:

- A good way to start to tell someone: "I have some important news to tell you."
- Do not tell anyone you have cancer while you are driving. It may be hard as people reach out to you once they find out, but try to avoid this. On the phone while driving, your emotions may sneak up on you. Pull over. Better yet, ask to call them back when you aren't driving.
- Tell people whatever you are comfortable sharing.
- You don't have to tell anyone everything all at once, especially younger children. Small doses over time can make it easier for them to understand and accept.
- When telling anyone, write down your bullet points of what you want to say. Telling people you love that you are ill can be hard. It can help to have your thoughts in writing, so you cover all you want to say.
- If people interrupt you while you are telling them about your diagnosis, it's okay to ask them to let you finish what you must say and after that they can ask all the questions they want.
- When you tell some people, they will insist on wanting to see you. If you like to be surrounded by people, then by all means do that! In the beginning, there is such a flurry of activity, you may feel like you are playing every position on the field at once and you are the only batter on the roster, or you may just want to be alone to process things. Some people will understand. Some will not. Don't let anyone guilt you into doing something you are not up to.
- If anyone offers to bring you meals, do not hesitate to tell them if you have any dietary restrictions, have chosen to make changes in your eating regimen, or there are things you have become sensitive to during your treatment.
- Do not be surprised if people say some incredibly silly or insensitive things when they find out.
- When telling your children, consider their age to determine how candid to be. You would explain how a

helicopter works far differently to a 20-year-old than you would a 3-year-old. This is the case with your illness, as well. If uncertain about how to tell your little ones, there are many books you can refer to with great suggestions or you can ask your doctor, nurse, or a social worker for advice in this area.

- Regardless of their age, ALL kids, in my experience, have the same two questions: Will I catch it? Are you going to die? Answer honestly and appropriately for their ages.
- After you tell your small children, it helps to ask them what they think caused the cancer so that you can dismiss the idea that they may have had anything to do with causing it. Small children are egocentric; the world revolves around them. Better to clear it up before it becomes a thought in their mind.
- I believe that our friends are incredibly well-meaning. With that being said, they may inundate you with alternative treatment suggestions, books they think you should read, movies about why this therapy is a rip off and only puts money in your doctor's pockets, or any other variety of things. I found that the best way to reply to these friends (some who may be quite forceful with their opinions of what THEY think your treatment should be) was to say, "Thank you for this information, but I have very carefully chosen my treatment path."

• • •

My story:

Prior to the call from Dr. Breast Surgeon telling me that the cancer might be far more extensive than first thought, we had decided to tell our children, one 24 and the other one 21 at the time of my diagnosis. I wanted to do it face to face. Or as face to face as you can when one of your children lives in New York. We kept it upbeat. Why not — this was all going to be easy peasy, right? Lumpectomy and five days of radiation.

Both kids were in very rigorous college programs, and I wanted this diagnosis to not impact what they were up to. I was incredibly worried that this might somehow derail them, or would negatively impact their grades at school. My intention was to make sure it didn't.

Since he lives near us, we first told our son, John; at the time a junior in Computer Engineering at Arizona State University. His response was just as I expected. He assured me I would be fine; that we had several friends who had survived breast cancer and they were all fine. And on that account, he was correct. (At least at that time.)

Our daughter, Landry, was attending The Pratt Institute in Brooklyn. Hubby had, weeks previously, planned a short trip, for some father/daughter time before school started for her, so he was already scheduled to see her. (Lucky Lows!) We decided that with him there we would tell her together over Skype. That way he was there to answer any questions (not that we had that many answers) and to be her support should she need it.

On the night he arrived, via technology, we shared the news with her. I vaguely remember the conversation, pretty much exactly what we had told our son the day before, with the additional information I had learned from Dr. Breast Surgeon given I had seen him that day. We talked about the genetic testing and that Dr. Breast Surgeon wanted an MRI before we went much further, and that he was having me see a radiation oncologist. She is her mother's daughter, so she was stoic, optimistic, and we were quickly making jokes about it. Yet, I felt very happy that Hubby was there with her.

On my end, with Hubby out of town, I was still shuttling Mom and FIL to doctor appointments. And wouldn't you know it, FIL became ill with a very bad cold on top of his heart problems.

Then my mom caught a cold as well.

[SHIT!!!!!]

As if that wasn't enough, a couple days into his visit, Hubby called to tell me that Landry woke up very ill. Temperature of 103 degrees and was delirious. I felt helpless as I tried to manage her insurance, find a doctor, and get them an appointment while trying to keep my brain from exploding from 2100 miles away. Moms are supposed to be with their children when they are sick. For the first time it felt like it pretty much sucked to be me right about then.

And the truth was, I was actually barely holding on, and knew I couldn't tell anyone as I'm always the strong one. I was holding on, however, my knuckles were getting very white and my palms were getting sweaty and slippery. I felt like I was quickly losing my grip on the bat.

The next calls I received were from Dr. Breast Surgeon with the date and time for my MRI and from the hospital confirming my MRI and . . . what a surprise . . . asking for money. Time to earn some flight miles.

Between shuttling Mom and FIL to appointments, I also had the BRCA testing and the MRI.

Once Dr. Breast Surgeon received the report from the MRI and the pathology report from the original biopsy, he scheduled with the hospital for another MRI with guided needle biopsy and an appointment with two new team members, Dr. Medical Oncologist and Dr. Plastic Surgeon.

Chemotherapy Treatment

Earlier, I shared that before I had it, I knew very little about cancer. What I knew about chemotherapy was even less.

I thought if you had cancer, you got chemo. Wrong.

I thought ALL chemo made you sick. Wrong again.

I thought everyone who had chemo lost their hair. Nope.

I thought all chemo was given IV or through a port. Wrong, yet again.

Unlike surgery and radiation, which target a specific part of the body, chemotherapy targets the whole body. Chemotherapy (aka chemo) can be given as the main treatment for some certain cancers, but more often it used with surgery and/or radiation.

Cancer cells grow more quickly than healthy cells; chemo drugs are designed to kill these fast-growing cells. As the chemo drug travels throughout the body, it may damage or destroy normal, healthy cells that are fast-growing as well, such as skin, hair, lining of the stomach, intestines, and bone marrow.

Most chemo drugs are given by pill, liquid you swallow, a shot, or in your vein, either through a needle in your arm or a venous port.

A port is a small disc made of metal or plastic. It is about the size of a quarter that is placed under your skin, usually somewhere on your chest, as an outpatient surgical procedure. Attached to the disc is small plastic flexible tube, called a catheter, that connects the port to a large vein.

Depending on your type and stage of cancer, and the drugs your doctor is using, you might receive chemo once a day, once a week, once every 10 days, or even once a month for several months to a year. Chemo is usually given in "cycles" with rest periods in between. In most cases the number of cycles you get depends on which drugs you are receiving for what type of cancer you have. The rest period between cycles allows normal cells to recover and your body to regain its strength. Sometimes your body needs additional time to return to normal, so your cycle may be delayed, adjustments made to the strength of the drugs, or the time between is even extended.

Chemo has gotten kinder and gentler over the years. Some people feel fine and continue to take care of things at home, can exercise, spend time with family and friends, and continue to work. But chemo drugs are still strong, so side effects can still occur. These are caused by the chemo's effect on healthy cells. For most people, side effects diminish over time between each cycle and go away over time after chemo ends. Some side effects take longer than others to go away and some might not go away at all.

One of the most important side effects of chemo is its effect on your blood cells. Blood cells are some of the fastest dividing cells in the body, making them the most sensitive to chemo. During your chemo, your doctor will keep track of your blood cell counts to assess how your body is tolerating the treatment.

While you are having chemotherapy, you will have your blood work drawn frequently and that becomes part of the treatment routine. Blood tests are usually done right before you get your chemo treatment to make sure your cell count is such that you can tolerate a treatment, and then a week or two later. These results help your doctor determine potential changes, if any, that might need to be made to your treatment.

Chemo drugs often stop the bone marrow from making enough blood cells. If your white blood cell count is low, you are more susceptible to infections. If your red blood cell counts are low, you may feel tired. If your platelets are low, you may bruise easily. If your blood counts fall below your normal range, your doctor might prescribe a medicine that stimulates your bone marrow to produce more white blood cells. These are supportive medications and do not treat your cancer. These medications are generally given as shots, usually 24 hours after a chemo treatment.

Just like with your other doctors, you will be interviewing your medical oncologist as well. And just like with all your other doctors, you will want to make sure you feel comfortable with this physician, as they may be the doctor you see the most often for the longest period.

You may want to ask some of the following questions before you decide to draft your medical oncologist for treatment:

> What is my diagnosis?
> What Stage is my cancer?
> What are my treatment options? What are the benefits of each option? What are the side effects?
> Should I undergo genetic testing?
> Will I need any additional testing?
> What is the test for?
> What will the results of the additional testing tell you?
> When will you get the results? How will I be informed?

- Do I need chemotherapy? Why?
- What is the goal of chemotherapy?
- What are the benefits?
- What are the chances it will work?
- How often is this chemotherapy performed for my type of cancer?
- How many times have you prescribed this treatment?
- What is your success rate?
- What are the possible complications, risks or side effects?
- Why do I need this treatment?
- Do I have cancer in my lymph nodes?
- What is the significance of cancer found in the lymph nodes?
- Are there any other alternatives to chemotherapy for my cancer?
- Will I need other cancer treatments, like surgery or radiation, before or after chemo?
- What will happen if I don't have chemo?
- What do I have to lose or gain if I don't have chemo?
- Am I healthy enough to have chemo?
- Are you certified by any Specialty Oncology Board?
- Will the chemo cure the cancer?
- How will I know the chemo is working?
- How many chemotherapy drugs will I get?
- How long will the chemo treatment take each time?
- How often?
- What happens if I get an infection?
- Will I need blood transfusions?
- Do I need a port?
- Do I need to do anything special to prepare for chemo?
- How will my chemo be given?
- How many treatments?
- Will I have to stay in the hospital? If so, how long?
- What happens if the chemo doesn't work?
- What can I expect after chemo? Will there be a lot of pain? Will I have any catheters coming out of my body?

- Can I sleep on my back, side, or stomach?
- How soon can I shower after the port is put in?
- Do I have any restrictions and if so, what are they and for how long?
- How will my body be affected by the chemo? Will it look or work differently? Will any of the changes be permanent?
- Will I be taking medicines after chemo? How do you spell it? How will I take it?
- What are the side effects?
- What are the chances my chemo will cause nausea and/or vomiting? If so, how long will it last?
- Which side effects should I report to you?
- Are there any medications I can take to prevent or treat side effects?
- Will this/these chemo drugs be okay to take with my other medicines?
- Can I drive to my treatments?
- Can I work during chemo? If not, how soon can I go back to work?
- Do I need to change my daily routine?
- How long before I can go back to my usual activities like the gym?
- What about sex?
- Do I have time to think about the other options or get a second opinion?
- How quickly must I decide about my treatment?
- Do I need to see my dentist before we start treatment?
- When should I begin?
- Will a delay in treatment reduce my chance of being cured?
- If I choose surveillance or the cancer comes back, how will I be treated?
- What is the percentage rate of developing a secondary cancer due to the chemotherapy treatment?
- What number should I call in an emergency?

➢ What is the name of the person I should communicate with in your office? Do they have a direct number?

These last two questions are usually addressed with the person responsible for billing:

➢ Will my insurance pay for this treatment?
➢ How much will my portion be?

You should never leave the medical oncologist's appointment with unanswered questions, unless they are about tests or pathology results that have not yet been completed.

It may help to know that your doctor wants you to know everything about your treatment and for you to fully understand it. Don't leave your initial visit with the medical oncologist without having all your questions answered.

You want the best oncologist, for you, as this will be a significant portion of your life for the next few months. You will want to be comfortable with the doctor, their support staff, and the infusion center. Do not rush, or feel rushed, during your initial visit. This is YOUR time to see if you feel comfortable with this person who will be caring for you for the next several months.

• • •

Tips:

- Take your 3-ring binder to the visits with the oncologist.
- Take someone with you or record the visit.
- Transfer your notes into your 3-ring binder.
- Copy the above questions or download them from www.holycrapihavecancer.com. Prior to your visit, cross

out the questions you already have answers to, so you can just concentrate on the ones you need answered.

- Even if you like the oncologist you have been referred to, do not hesitate to get a second opinion on their treatment recommendation to ease any concerns you might have that there could be other options. This journey belongs to no one but you.
- Every person tolerates chemotherapy differently. You could get the exact same drugs as another person and have no side effects, while the other person gets them all. Don't get caught up in the comparison game. (I did. I hated that I couldn't drive myself to and from chemo, but I had all these other friends that could. The little voice in my head HATED it.)
- If you are getting your chemo through an IV or port, chemo day can last anywhere from a few hours to most of the day. You can read, listen to music, visit with friends, make new friends, do crafts or play games. Bring the activities you like, to help pass the time.
- If you have a port, you will be prescribed a numbing cream (if not prescribed – ask for it) to use the day of your treatment. Be generous with the cream one hour before your appointment. Use a big glob! Cover with a square of "Glad Press and Seal" to keep the glob in place and to protect your clothing.
- Most infusion centers have blankets available that are washed daily; but don't hesitate to take your own if you have one you love or if someone made you a special chemo blanket.
- Stay hydrated before, during and after treatment.
- Pre-chemo jitters are not unusual. (Beginning with my second cycle, once my son drove away, I would puke in the garbage can in the parking lot before each treatment.) My oncology nurse shared that it was not unusual to have pre-chemo anxiety and nausea.

- Take snacks or a meal. Or let one of your support team bring you lunch mid-day, if you are going to be there for the entire day. It breaks up the day for you and allows them to contribute.
- If you have time before you start treatment, get your teeth cleaned. You may not be able to get them cleaned during chemo and it's possible the chemo will give you mouth sores. Starting with a freshly clean
- mouth helps. Brush frequently with a very soft toothbrush. You can brush with baking soda, rinse with baking soda, and saltwater gargles helps as well. There is also a mild mouthwash called Biotene that works well. If you get sores, be sure to tell your team. If the sores get unmanageable, talk with your physician as there are prescriptions available to help.
- Some people lose weight during chemo due to the nausea and decreased appetite and some people gain weight due to the reduction in activity and sometimes frequent use of crackers and bread to decrease symptoms of nausea. The time to worry about your weight is after active treatment is over, unless your Oncologist gets concerned about you losing too much weight. They will come up with a plan should that happen.
- If you are considering a wig, get it before chemo when you still feel up to picking it out. Have fun. Always wanted to be a redhead? Now is your opportunity. Embrace it. I have seen women's personality blossom when they had fun with their wigs.
- Get a fleece or soft beanie if you will be losing your hair. You will quickly realize you've been wearing a hair hat your whole life. Now you will need a real one since your hair growth is on temporary hiatus. You may find you also need a thin, soft beanie to wear at night as your uncovered head may get cold. You can find these online.

- Some people find relief with ginger. Ginger teas, pieces of fresh ginger or even ginger lozenges or gum which can be found in health food stores or online.
- Don't be surprised that after chemo your brain just kind of doesn't work very well for a few days. I couldn't read or track a television program those first few days after chemo. My patio swing was my respite on those days.
- This is one of those side effects that can linger even after your chemo treatment is completed.
- Chemo brain is real!!! Chemo brain can start during or after your treatment. Doctors don't fully understand why you get chemo brain. Some studies show that chemotherapy slows the growth of cells in areas of the brain that handle things like learning and memory. Some researchers think other things contribute as well. The symptoms of chemo brain may disappear quickly after your chemotherapy ends, or they may linger for months. What I can tell you is chemo brain is a real thing.
- Long term treatment can lead to depression and anxiety. Do not be afraid to share with your doctor any mental changes you may have, as they can be dealt with while you are going through treatment. There is no reason to white-knuckle it. Of the hundreds of survivors I have spoken with or met, I have yet to meet one, who had extended treatment, who didn't have medication of some kind, at some point, for the anxiety or depression.
- Chemotherapy can cause vaginal dryness which can be a problem during and after treatments. There are many products that can alleviate the problem such as lubricants available at your pharmacy, intimate product retail store or online. Do not hesitate to discuss with your doctor or nurse practitioner if your situation does not improve as there are medical therapies as well.
- Discuss the impact of your treatment with your employer. Some workplaces may allow you to work flexible hours during or after chemotherapy. Some may provide you a

place to rest during the day. Openly discuss your situation with your employer if you are in a smaller business, or your Human Resources representative if you are employed by a larger company.

Ann's Tips:

- I found that ice chips and or popsicles **DURING** chemotherapy helped to reduce the mouth sores. I didn't do it on the first cycle and suffered for weeks with sores. I did this with the rest of my cycles and experienced only minor mouth sores, or none at all.
- Stay hydrated. As time went on and my chemo brain got worse, I got terrible about remembering how much water I had consumed. I kept a glass bottle, filled with room temperature water on my counter. (I found I could tolerate room temperature water better than cold water.) I placed 8 hair rubber bands (I certainly didn't need them anymore!) around the bottle. Each morning I rolled those to the bottom of the bottle and as I consumed the entire bottle of water, I would roll a hair band up to the top of the bottle. This helped me remind myself to stay hydrated and, as my chemo brain increased, it helped me to keep track of the amount I had consumed as sometimes it was easy to forget. There are also water bottles available online to remind you to drink throughout the day.
- My Oncologist said that the shot the day after chemo to raise my white blood cell count might feel like growing pains if you had those growing up. If you are one of the fortunate individuals that did not experience them as a child, they are cramping muscle aches and bone pains that occur in some children. Your Oncologist may have you using something to prevent or decrease the side effects. I was instructed to use Claritin and Aleve and

found that using it for **5 full days** after the shot helped reduce the bone and joint pain.

- Some days the Claritin and Aleve just weren't enough. This bath remedy relieved some of the ache as well and I found myself doing it multiple times a day on the worst days:
  o One cup of Epsom Salt
  o One cup of baking soda, and
  o 10 drops of a high-quality essential oil. Use only premium quality essential oils that are Certified Pure Therapeutic Grade so you know you are getting the purest products available as they will be absorbed through your skin.
- Chemo dries your skin. I tried many different lotions and finally was gifted, by one of my body workers, a recipe of something that worked best for me that I called my Love Potion. (I still use it today!) One-part Organic Olive Oil, one-part Organic Coconut Oil and 1/3-part Organic Avocado Oil all mixed together in one large glass container. (I bought all the oils at Costco and I used a 32-ounce glass bottle with a stopper which you can easily find on Amazon.) Depending on the amount you mix at one time, add anywhere from a few drops to two bottles of an essential oil. I added doTERRA On Guard but there are many essential oils that provide immune support, just make sure it is a therapeutic grade essential oil. I mixed a 32-ounce batch, as I didn't want to have to be mixing it frequently, and poured it into a smaller bottle that I kept handy. Both bottles also received a giant LOVE sticker on them so that every time I used it I pictured covering my body with LOVE. Chemo is tough, and your body needs as much love as possible.
- Add one or two drops of an immunity support essential oil to your facial moisturizer. The further I got into my chemo, the lower my blood counts got, the more fearful I became of getting ill – not chemo ill, but flu or cold ill,

on top of chemo ill. I was frequently exposed to colds and flu at doctor's appointments and yet I never caught anything. I'm not sure it was the frequent use of the immunity boosting essential oil, but I was the only person I knew of using it and the only one who did not catch some other virus during chemo.

- I listened to the Chemotherapy Mediation from Breethe by OMG I Can Mediate when I had chemotherapy. Many other meditation apps now also have chemotherapy meditations. Research the meditation apps available for your smartphone as there are many available and probably have cancer meditations.
- Every day when I would shower, I would visualize the dying cancer cells being washed down the drain. It was just my proactive way of visualizing the cancer leaving my body.
- There is very little you have control over during this time except your attitude. Attitude still makes a difference in life; especially with cancer. When things get difficult, put the biggest smile on your face – even if it feels fake. A smile – even a fake one — can shift how you actually feel.
- Stick to only happy and upbeat TV shows, movies and books. I "un-friended" people who were negative and seemed to have nothing but drama in their life. I couldn't have that kind of energy in my life during that time. It ended up being so healthy for me, I actually still continue to do the same thing to this day. Cancer left me in a different place with no room for drama or negativity.
- Sleep. I was an insomniac since my pre-teens. I felt I had a good night's slumber if I got 4 or 5 hours of shut-eye nightly. I had known for years that my sleep patterns were not good for my health or my weight. I used this time to retrain my body to get plenty of sleep. You may require a prescription for a sleeping pill, but do whatever you can to get at least 8 – 10 hours of sleep. Your body

is going through a lot. Give it plenty of opportunities to heal by getting at least 8 hours of sleep per day.

- Eat whatever you feel like, unless you decide that this is your opportunity to make healthy lifestyle changes or you follow the science of the benefits of a ketogenic diet for cancer and during chemotherapy. I started with the best of intentions of eating only healthy foods, but there were times that the only thing that tasted good and would stay down was my favorite smoothie. Small frequent meals are better than large, heavy, meals. However, if you are a person that can make these lifestyle changes at this time, there is a growing amount of scientific benefit to the positive for fasting prior to chemotherapy, and for chemotherapy responding better if the patient is adhering to a ketogenic diet during chemotherapy.

- If you will receive a chemotherapy agent that will cause you to lose your hair, you may or may not also lose hair from your eyebrows, eyelashes, arms, legs chest and pubic region. I'm not sure why I didn't think about it before, (I guess you don't have to be very smart to get cancer.) but I also lost the hairs inside my nose. It isn't a concern other than it can cause your nose to run A LOT and you lose your first line of defense against germs. I also quickly learned that my hair was an incredible feeler preventing me from bashing my head against open cabinets, tree limbs or an array of other low hanging objects. If you lose your hair be prepared to bonk your head until you get used to being aware of your surroundings so you don't knock yourself silly.

- If you do not use some form of electronic calendar, use the one in your three-ring binder to keep track of appointments, social commitments and any other important events like birthdays (No, the world doesn't stop because you have cancer. Life keeps lifing.)

- Exercise. I know I keep saying this. It had such a positive impact on me, I think it is worth mentioning frequently.

Now is not the time to start training for a marathon, but taking a walk for as long as you can tolerate helps increase your energy, clear your mind, helps relieve constipation and can help you sleep better. Search for walking meditations or listen to your favorite music or books on apps like Audible. Otherwise, if you are anything like me YOUR little voice in your head might put YOU on the crazy train.)

- If you are in one of the 29 states or Washington D.C (as of 11/2017) that allows the use of Medical Marijuana, consider getting a Medical Marijuana card. The marijuana today is not your mother's or father's marijuana. Today's marijuana comes in a variety of forms with strengths that are measured and controlled: buds to inhale by smoking or vaporizing, tinctures and edibles. It also comes in different types: Sativa – which is better for during the day and when you need to be awake or Indica which is good if you need to really relax or sleep. You can also find products that do not contain the main psychoactive compound (THC) known as CBD's. Marijuana can reduce nausea and vomiting, improve food intake, can reduce pain, and can improve sleep. Smoking or vaping will give you more immediate results, where edibles effects take longer to notice but will last several hours. As with any recommendation in this book, confirm its usage with your physicians first. Your physicians may even be able to write you the necessary prescription to provide for the application for the Medical Marijuana card registry process or you may have to go to a physician that specifically does exams for you to apply for a card. (Google your state to find out the current laws, what is required to qualify for a medical marijuana card and how to apply.)
- Consider starting turmeric. The benefits have been well documented in medical literature that turmeric and curcumin, one of the bioactive ingredients in turmeric,

have been found to promote health and protect against a wide variety of health conditions. Because of these studies (with many more ongoing), it has been shown that curcumin can benefit your health in a variety of ways. My oncologist recommended I start turmeric and I'm glad I did. I tried several varieties, but I have always have gone back to Doctor's Best Curcumin Phytosome that can be purchased at many vitamin shops, Sprouts, Whole Foods or on Amazon. (If purchasing this online at Amazon make sure it comes from the Doctor's Best Amazon store or go directly to their website: www.drbvitamins.com to assure the quality of the product. Unfortunately, the sales of vitamins and supplements online has become wrought with fraud, so you will want to make sure you are getting them from a reliable source.

- I didn't do this, but I wish I had: I met a survivor who wore the same outfit to each chemotherapy treatment and when she was done, she ceremoniously burned them. Cancer is filled with little milestones. I found ceremonies pretty enjoyable – like throwing out my sheets, t-shirts and bras after radiation. These ceremonies were a mark of progress for me. I would encourage you to find your own ceremonies that inspire you.

• • •

My Story:

Dr. Breast Surgeon called me on August 20. He was right; we were quickly becoming breast friends. At this rate we would be planning a family vacation together...me and Mrs. Dr. Breast Surgeon walking on the beach each morning while Hubby and Dr. Breast Surgeon sat in lounge chairs, pretending to watch

the waves rather than the scantily clad volleyball players. . . .
WHOA...come away from the light, Ann. You've gone too far.

But it did seem like I was hearing from him frequently. This
call was Dr. Breast Surgeon calling to tell me he had received
the report on my BRCA testing and it had come back negative.
Well. . . whattya know. . . finally something positive.
I really was extremely relieved as I wasn't sure I was up for a
conversation about cutting out my lower lady parts when I
was already considering having both girls removed. At least
not yet!

He also said that he had spoken to Dr. Medical Oncologist, and
Dr. Medical Oncologist wanted me to have a PET scan before
we were to meet for the first time, since the original MRI
suggested lymph node involvement.

It was actually reassuring to know I was getting a PET scan. I
knew enough that a PET scan would show if the cancer had
spread to anywhere else in my body. It felt to me like it would
be the definitive closure of all the information we needed for
Ann's Cancer. With a PET scan, we would have enough
information to know the recommended path with some
certainty.

Dr. Breast Surgeon also still wanted me to meet with Dr.
Plastic Surgeon since we now knew there was possibly going
to be some reconstruction involved. He figured it was best to
at least have a conversation with Dr. Plastic Surgeon, given
that I was no longer a candidate for a lumpectomy, so I could
better make my decision about what I was going to do.
Mastectomy? Double mastectomy? Reconstruction? No
reconstruction?

So many decisions!

Fortunately, I had some time.

Handsome and friendly, I was fortunate to like Dr. Plastic Surgeon immediately. I'd heard such horror stories from others about their awful first-time appointments, discomfort with their doctors and ongoing negative sagas with various doctors, that I was pretty sure that the good fortune of the Lucky Lows was smiling down upon on us.

I had, for years, always said that if I ever was diagnosed with breast cancer I would just lop them off. But now faced with really HAVING to make the decision, it didn't come as easily as I thought it would. I was actually having a hard time with my decision. I only had cancer in one breast and I was struggling with removing something that was, at that point, healthy. But I also knew I only wanted to do this once.

My first meeting with Dr. Plastic Surgeon was just information gathering. I was still collecting information to try and formulate my game plan. Like all of this, I knew little, or next to nothing, about the process of breast reconstruction after a mastectomy. When he told me that reconstruction was a total of up to four different surgeries, I almost fell off the table. Remember, I still had this crazy, and what was now proving to be unrealistic, notion I would get this all done before the end of the year. Four surgeries and time to heal in-between was definitely NOT going to allow for that to occur.

[SHIT. SHIT. SHIT. SHIT!]

Then there was the OBVIOUS fact that if I had a mastectomy on just the one side, I had another extremely large, floppy breast that he was going to have to attempt to match, which he said he would do his best accomplish, but given my natural size I would likely always have a pretty obvious difference.

My breasticles were, again, a problem.

I would be lying if I said I didn't waffle back and forth nearly every day about whether to remove just the one or to remove both breasts. Fortunately, with chemotherapy on my agenda first, I had time to think about it, ask others, and then consider my decision.

And waffle back and forth.

Eight days after my call from Dr. Breast Surgeon I had a PET scan; five days later, I had the MRI–guided needle biopsy (gotta find out if those newly discovered tumors are really cancerous); and the day after the second MRI, I had my first visit with Dr. Medical Oncologist.

A little slight in stature, impeccably dressed and fit, he breezed into the room with a three-ring binder under his arm.

He introduced himself and asked how I was. I replied like I always do, "Awesome!" With a surprised look on his face he said, "I don't usually get that kind of response on a first visit." I responded, "So far, I know I'm in great hands, so why be anything but awesome?"

I truly believed I was in good hands and I had accepted that I had cancer, so I was ready to take it on. And at the end of THIS visit, I knew I was going to know the plan. All the poking, squishing, pulling, jabbing, prodding, nudging, and bloodletting were now all going to fit together, like puzzle pieces, to paint the picture of Ann's Cancer and what we were going to do about it.

In that three-ring binder he held under his arm was ME. Everything that had been collected about me thus far. Mammogram results. Biopsy results. MRI results. Pet scan results. BRCA results. There was something about seeing him walk in with a three-ring binder, instead of the old regular doctor's chart, that bothered me more than I would have thought. Having been in clinical medicine for most of my working career, I always knew the sicker the patient the thicker the chart. This seemed like a scary start and left me feeling incredibly unsettled.

Up to this point I knew I had cancer and I knew I would be able to push myself through it; just like I had done with everything my entire life. (They don't call me Jane Wayne - the female version of John Wayne -for no reason.) For the first time, I wondered if I might not be able to just push myself through this.

*For the first time, it **really** struck me, no matter how unchanged I felt or currently looked in the mirror . . . **I was sick**.*

Once we got past the pleasantries, he began to tell me about my specific cancer. He drew a little picture of a cancer cell when it is considered "in situ." That means that the cancer is in an early stage and the growth, or tumor, is still confined to the site where the cancer started. He then drew a new picture showing how the cancer can escape and invade neighboring tissues and enter nearby lymph nodes or spread to other areas. He told me that the PET scan results indicated that my cancer had indeed spread to my lymph nodes.

*Oh, **AND** unrelated to the breast cancer, I had a spot that lit up on my colon, so I needed to have a colonoscopy as soon as possible to rule out colon cancer.*

WHAT!!??

As I recovered from that gut punch, he explained my diagnosis. I had Stage 3, Grade 3, Triple Positive Invasive Ductal Carcinoma. Then he said something that took the wind right out of my sails. He said that I was lucky that I had this diagnosis now because of the advancement of new treatment options, as five years ago, someone with this diagnosis only had a 15 percent survival rate at five years.

That three-ring binder. Five-year survival. 15 percent. Lucky? If he had tapped on the top of my head and said, "Helloooo, anyone in there?" there would have just been that hollow thud of the sound of something empty.

Now feeling pretty proud of myself (sarcasm font) that I had come to this appointment by myself because I was now overwhelmed and only halfway present, I vaguely listened as he then told me that I needed chemotherapy.

However odd I was in that moment, he was wonderful. Thorough. Clear. Descriptive. Concise. Sensible. Easy to understand. He didn't talk over my head and was matter-of-fact about it such that I felt comfortable with him and well informed.

What he did tell me, bluntly, was that I would lose my hair, I would probably not feel well, but would be given medications to aid in controlling that as much as possible and that I would have constipation and/or diarrhea — not in any particular order, but probably both as everybody reacts differently to the different chemotherapy drugs.

[Oh SHIT!! Literally!]

He recommended that I have a chemo port put in, given that I was going to be having chemo for six months, and a full year of a drug called Herceptin. He also told me that there was another new medication, called Perjeta, that he would be using. But that for now it was only approved by my insurance to be used prior to surgery, so we would start chemo as soon as I could have the port placed and surgery would be down the road after active chemotherapy was completed.

[WHOA, WHOA, WHOA!!! Hold up there! A year? ??Did he not get the memo about me NEEDING to have this all done by the end of the year? This is not going as I expected!]

The hits just kept right on coming as he told me that Perjeta and Herceptin each have the potential to cause congestive heart failure so I would need to have a baseline echocardiogram before we started, and I would be having several of them during my year of Herceptin. He wanted to arrange to have that done as quickly as possible.

He also gave me the name of the gastroenterologist to go see for the spot on my colon. When I asked him how soon I needed to schedule THAT appointment he replied, "I wouldn't wait."

[WHAAAT?!!!!]

"You mean during all of this?"

"Yes."

Just another day and another huge kick in the ovaries. Couldn't I just go back to the lumpectomy and five days of radiation?

At the time, I still wasn't certain what I was going to do about my breasticles. Dr. Breast Surgeon was a proponent of breast conservation and yet Dr. Plastic Surgeon articulated that he was going to have a hard time matching new perky girl, with an existing saggy double D. I shared with Dr. Medical Oncologist that I just wasn't sure what to do to which he replied, "Let me help you a little bit with that decision." 1) I may not have tested positive for the BRCA mutations, but he felt that with such a strong family history, there was definitely some type of genetic flaw that, probably, someday down the road would be isolated and identified. 2) I was only 53 which is considered young for cancer. 3) I had very dense breasts. 4) I had an aggressive type of cancer. For those four reasons, he recommended I have a double mastectomy.

After that he introduced me to his Nurse Practitioner. Friendly, knowledgeable, and kind, she seemed genuinely concerned. I instantly felt at ease with her and knew I would feel comfortable in her capable hands as well.

With my appointment with Dr. Gastroenterologist on the books for the first available opening on September 15, my mind made up about what type of surgery I was having, an echocardiogram scheduled in two days, and after the echocardiogram — later that same day — scheduled return to Dr. Medical Oncologist's office for what I called "Chemo Camp," I drove home, my dropped jaw still resting on my chest. A year of infusions? Colon cancer? Double mastectomy? Colonoscopy?

It all seemed too much too soon. To say the least, I was overwhelmed.

After talking to hundreds of cancer patients and survivors, I have found that for as many different practices as there are out there, there seems to be that many ways they go over your treatment plan in detail. In this practice, they have you return to the office prior to the first cycle and you are required to bring your main caregiver so they fully understand things as well

After the echocardiogram, with Hubby in tow for his first doctor's visit with me so far, off we went to "Chemo Camp." We were called back to a room with a video player and TV where we me, Ms. Oncology Nurse who had us watch a video that was a basic overview of cancer and chemotherapy. It explained some side effects and briefly covered what to expect; it even talked about sex.

[Oh SHIT. Sex??? I hadn't given that any thought for weeks. Poor Hubby.]

Good thing the video pointed out that if there wasn't a lack of sex right now, it probably would happen during chemotherapy.

[Oh Goodie. More chaos for my already messed-up mind.]

She gave me a folder...not just a few papers...a thick fucking folder full of information about the different drugs and their possible side effects, information to prepare for what was upcoming and all the possible practice contact information I could possibly need. I was eventually grateful for that folder, but at the time I was becoming more overwhelmed. No, not true. I was getting scared. She went over the four chemo drugs I would be getting.

[FOUR of them????]

She then got more specific about the side effects — nausea, vomiting, mouth sores, neuropathy — temporary, but could be permanent.

[Wow, this sounds fun!]

Diarrhea, fatigue, low white cell counts. Anemia, constipation, hair loss.

[This just keeps getting better and better. Can we start today?]

She reviewed the instructions I was to follow pre-infusion and the routine for medications after the treatment.

[One pill makes you larger, And one pill makes you small. And the ones that Mother gives you don't do anything at all...Go ask Alice, when she's ten feet tall.]

144

She went over the shot I would receive the day after each chemo treatment, and its side effects.

[More side effects? Really? This sounds so enjoyable – what the hell ARE we waiting for?]

She provided a list of over-the-counter medications that would be beneficial to have on hand. (She was right; I used every one of them.) She reviewed instructions of my prescribed and over-the-counter medications I was to start taking before my first infusion and what to take after. She gave me hand-outs on how to manage the different side effects, where I could get a wig, websites where I could get TRUSTED information, recommended reading material, information on support groups. . . .

[NOPE – not for this cowgirl!]

and the numbers to call if I had any questions or an emergency.

[Emergency? There can be emergencies?]

She finished by telling me that, because of the drugs I was going to be given prior to each infusion to diminish side effects during the infusion . . . .

[side effects DURING the infusion???]

. . . . I wouldn't be able to drive myself to or from my chemo treatments. I was beginning to feel more and more like I had lost any control I had over my life.

I was not a happy camper! For some reason my fear was suddenly replaced with anger. **Inside I was pissed!** I'm not sure what I was expecting, but for some reason it was making me mad, which in looking back now seems very strange but it *just shows that this journey will have you all over the place emotionally.*

Then...drum roll please...it was time to go back to see Dr. Medical Oncologist to get any last questions answered and to find out how many weeks I had to get my shit together before we started all of this.

I often kid frequently that I'm spontaneous as long as I have a couple weeks to plan for it; so far things had been happening pretty quickly and I felt I had a lot of things I needed to complete before I was ready to start ANYTHING. I was still shuttling Mom and FIL to therapy treatments or doctor appointments as well as running a business.

I needed time.

[Like a couple years. Or how about NEVER!]

Then Dr. Medical Oncologist had the audacity to tell us that he and Dr. Breast Surgeon had been communicating and I was scheduled to have the port placed the following Tuesday – only 4 days away – and I would have my first infusion of chemotherapy the following day, and every 21 days after that.

[WHAAT? Are you FUCKING KIDDING ME??? I have things to do. It would all start in 4 days??? NOOOO!!!]

This all seemed to be happening so fast that my head was spinning. Calm on the outside. Storm surge on the inside. The voice in my head was now going crazy, screaming at me to run. Get the hell out of there. I didn't run; but I sure felt like it. I wanted to run and keep on going. I felt like nothing was in my control and as someone who feels like I need to control things in order to stay on this planet, I was so uncomfortable that I felt like I could no longer stay in my skin suit.

I may have felt out of control, however, I was now fully equipped (like it or not) with my diagnosis, treatment plan, and all the information that I seemed to need for the year-long adventure that lay ahead of me. Even though I felt so discombobulated, I recognized a new feeling; I was now very nervous. But even with my brain in overdrive, the voice in my head screaming interjections, and my skin suit feeling 3 sizes too small, I felt pretty certain that with one foot in front of the other, everything was going to be turn out fine. Millions had gone before me and it was now my time to pay the dues to become a reluctant member of the cancer club.

Work and Cancer

A study by the National Coalition for Cancer Survivorship and Amgen, Inc., (published in the book *Handbook of Cancer Survivorship* by Michael Feuerstein, editor) states that 81 percent of cancer patients and survivors who participated in the study claimed that maintaining some semblance of a "normal" work routine provided emotional stability during the ups and downs of going through cancer treatment.

The employment concerns of cancer patients have changed dramatically since the 1970s when less than one-half of those diagnosed with cancer survived more than five years. (Yay modern medicine!)

A national survey of cancer survivors found that most employers tend to be sensitive, willing to help, and supportive to employees who have cancer.

Although the attitudes of cancer survivors, their co-workers, and their employers have changed over the years, it seems that most cancer survivors want to, and are able to, work during treatment and return to their jobs completely after treatment.

Your ability to keep your normal work schedule throughout treatment will depend on your diagnosis, treatment, and financial situation. You are generally not required to disclose anything about your diagnosis to your current employer unless you find that you need to take time off for treatment, or you might need some other considerations. In those cases, you will need to reveal some information about your medical condition to receive protection under the American Disabilities Act, The Family and Medical Leave Act of 1993, and the Genetic Information Nondiscrimination Act. (This information applies to the United States; you will need to investigate the laws, benefits, and social services available in your country of residence to find out what your rights are.)

There are many ways to work through your treatment or to give yourself a break if you need it. Should it come to needing to revise your schedule or take some necessary time off, talk with your employer to create a plan that supports everyone involved.

Flexible working hours or revised schedule: Under federal and state laws, some employers may be required to let you work a flexible schedule to meet your treatment needs. Explore the option of working from home, job sharing, or telecommuting.

Leave of absence: The Family Medical Leave Act of 1993 allows employees to leave work for up to 12 weeks for medical treatment and allows you to keep your benefits, without losing your job. While the leave is unpaid, taking it allows you to continue your health insurance for those 12 weeks. It can be taken all at once or as you need it. (This law only applies to employers with 50 or more employees, all government agencies, and schools nationwide. You must be a full-time employee and you must have been an employee of the company for at least a year.)

Short-term Disability: This program provides a percentage of your income in the case of an injury or illness that keeps you from working. Short-term disability may be granted by the state or the employers for a pre-determined time, usually three to six months.

• • •

Unfortunately, there is never a good time to get cancer and it is a very tough way to find out you don't control the world. The reality is that as much as you might like to control things and have your world operate as "business as usual," the reality is that over the next three to 12 months, maybe even longer, your cancer is going to take the place at the front of your kids, parents, work, and life in general. The extent of that will depend on your diagnosis and treatment.

• • •

Tips:

- Talk to your human resources department to find out what your company policies are and what you might be eligible for.
- Keep your employer-sponsored health insurance at all costs.
- Keep your supervisor up to date on how well (or not) your schedule or work arrangements are working for you. Renegotiate and make changes as you might need.
- Plan chemo treatments late in the day or right before the weekend to give you time to recover.
- If you can, get more help at home so you have more energy for work.
- Unless there is some reason you do not want them to know, let co-workers know about your situation. You may be incredibly surprised by the support you get and how many may be able to help you manage your work during this time.

- If you will be job sharing, make a detailed list of job duties so that others know how to handle things when you are out of the office.
- Don't hesitate to reconsider your decision to keep working if you find that working isn't going well for you. None of us know how we will feel during treatment; if you find you need to rethink your decision, do not hesitate to do that.
- If you live in a state that provides paid short-term disability leave (as of 2017 those states include California, New York, New Jersey, Hawaii, and Rhode Island), apply as soon as you know you will be taking a leave from work.
- Should your family need assistance with basic needs such as food and supplies, contact your local department of human services or welfare unit to apply for food stamps or other available programs you might qualify for. (www.acf.hhs.gov or call 877-696-6775.)
- There are other financial resources available to cancer patients. These usually have eligibility requirements based upon income and assets:
  - CancerCare: The American Society of Clinical Oncology has several different programs. Some cover the cost of cancer treatment; these are often earmarked for certain types of cancer. They also offer financial assistance to help patients pay for transportation, childcare, or even home care expenses. (http://www.cancercare.org/get_help/assistance/index.php)
  - American Cancer Society: Functions as more of a referral service. They offer information about many programs, both nationally and locally. There are programs that help with transportation, wigs, and other services. (www.cancer.org)

- o United Way: A clearinghouse to find programs offered nationally and locally. (http://www.liveunited.org)
  - o Supplemental Security Income (SSI): Federal income supplement program funded by general tax revenues not Social Security revenues. It is designed to assist the aged, blind, and disabled who have little or no income. It provides cash to meet basic needs for food, clothing, and shelter. (www.ssa.gov/disabilityssi)
- Investigate assistance for specific types of cancer. Many cancer organizations offer a variety of financial assistance programs that can cover co-pay assistance, transportation, home care, and child care. To find these organizations search the Internet by typing in your specific type of cancer and words like financial aid or financial assistance.
- Ask your doctors or other patients if they know of any organizations that offer assistance of some kind, or financial aid for patients in your situation.
- You will find a long list of resources at the end of this book that might assist you during this time.

• • •

My Story:

*There is something that is a part of my previous medical history that I was told I **always** needed to share with any my surgeons prior to having any surgical procedure. In 2009 I broke my ankle badly enough to require surgery. It wasn't the ankle fracture, hospitalization, surgery, or the eight weeks of no weight-bearing that was worthy of remembering, or even mattered with my current situation; it was the subsequent* staph infection, with its additional surgeries to clean the wound of infection, another week in the hospital, and 42 days of IV antibiotics, that was the consideration. When I saw Dr. Infectious Disease for the last time after all that treatment, he told me that I would **always** need to communicate to my doctors, any time I was to have ANY kind of surgery, that I was a "staph carrier," so that the surgeon would know to aggressively pre-treat me with antibiotics to prevent a recurrence of another staph infection. According to him I had an 85% risk of another infection whenever I had surgery.

So, at every appointment and in every document I completed, I let everyone (Dr. Biopsy, MRI Technician, the girl who called from the hospital for my history before the guided needle biopsy, Dr. Breast Surgeon, Dr. Plastic Surgeon, Dr. Radiation Oncologist, and Dr. Medical Oncologist, surgical nurse, anyone who would listen) know that I was a staph carrier. I wasn't afraid to look foolish by telling everyone; but I DEFINITELY did not want a repeat of my ankle infection as it was horrific. (I think English teachers and professional writers call this paragraph foreshadowing. If this were a movie, some dramatic music would begin playing in the background.)

Tuesday arrived way faster than I expected and, in what seemed like a blink of an eye, I was at the hospital to have the port placed.

Hubby dropped me off bright and early on the morning of September 9. He and I had an agreement: he was in charge of keeping our boat afloat; I was in charge of being the patient. We own a Commercial General Contracting business together and it functions on the basis of no work, no income. Him sitting for four or five hours in a waiting room, doing nothing, is an impractical business practice for us. Plus, I was in the best of hands: my breast friend, Dr. Breast Surgeon. And realistically, what was Hubby going to do if there was an emergency. . . rush into the operating room and perform CPR? Just the *thought of that makes me snicker out loud. Hubby, who is probably one of the most intelligent men I know, knows so little about medicine it makes me laugh a little to picture him contributing by doing life-saving measures.*

First, I was whizzing through the admissions process . . . ."We need your portion today, Mrs. Low."

[Here, accept my first born.]

Then I was getting in my lovely breezy gown, having an IV started, and answering the same questions I felt like I had answered 100 times already over the past few weeks, and then Dr. Breast Surgeon came briskly in. We exchanged the usual hellos, and then he said that he had just received the results of the guided needle biopsy that I'd had done exactly one week prior at this very same hospital.

[Pretty sure that was months ago.]

He informed me that the two tumors were not just pissed off spots; they had also come back as malignant. Always trying to find levity in EVERY situation, I said "So I guess this isn't where you tell me this has all been a cruel joke." He responded, "No, I'll see you in the operating room."

Wow. I had completely forgotten about those results. Everything had been moving so quickly, and I already knew I had an aggressive type of cancer, that confirming that the two tumors found on the MRI were malignant had pretty much totally slipped my mind.

My last memory was of the anesthesiologist saying. "Okay you might feel a little". . . . I have no recollection of recovery, talking to any of the doctors, or going home; but I obviously got there.

With the port securely placed between my breasts, a location I would come to loathe, the next day, having followed all my pre-chemo instructions, and loaded down with enough crap in a bag to keep me busy for months rather than the 6 hours I was scheduled to be there, I rode with my son, John, who dropped me off for my very first chemotherapy treatment.

"I'm fine. Just drop me off."

He insisted on walking me to the door. (I think he was actually just keeping an eye on me in case I decided to duck out and run.) But with fake bravado, we hugged, he went to his car and I entered into what would be my new home away from home, every week, for the next 52 weeks. I was checked in and led to the infusion room. This consisted of a very large room with a nurse's station in the center. There was activity all around; nurses bustling between patients and checking pumps and quantities in chemo bags. There was beeping followed by, "You're almost done." At least 10 other people were either in reclining chairs or walking around pushing their IV poles. A patient and her sister were at a table working on a jigsaw puzzle, while others were snuggled under blankets sleeping or just resting. Some were reading and some chatting with whomever was there with them. Some were alone and others had several people with them. Some looked like they weren't even sick and others looked, quite frankly, on death's door.

The place was packed and bustling with activity.

A nurse spotted me standing there with my overstuffed bag and what I suspect was a dumbass, stupefied, nervous, look on my face and she said, "We are a bit busy today. Usually, you can sit take any open chair, but right now there is only one empty spot over there. Why don't you get settled and a nurse will be right over."

Cocktail hour was about to begin.

Nurse Angel Girl came over, introduced herself, confirmed who I was, and verified my insurance. She started asking me a variety of questions: had I taken my steroids, did I understand what we were going to be doing today, did I bring anyone with me, did I need water? She showed me how to unplug my pump from the wall (in order to use the restroom or walk around) and the refrigerator filled with water and Ensure, the room where I could go in and watch television if I wanted, and the areas with magazines and puzzles. She recommended that I have a blanket and a pillow, as some of the pre-chemo drugs they would give me to decrease my chances of side effects would probably make me drowsy and perhaps chilly. She brought those over with the comment, "These are here if you need them; they are washed every night; but feel free to bring your own next time, if you would prefer."

[Oh yeah, next time. Shit!]

I may have been joking and trying to be humorous, like I always try to be, but I was already feeling anxious for Cycle 2 and I hadn't even had the first one yet.

She explained that, with the prep and the four drugs I was receiving, I would be there at least six hours, but longer if I started to have any negative reactions. If I did have a negative reaction, they would slow down how quickly the drugs were being infused and possibly give me additional medications to offset the reactions.

[Alright. I've changed my mind. I ABSOLUTLEY **DO NOT** want to do this!]

And then it was time. The moment of truth. She asked if I was ready and I told her that I was as ready as I was ever going to be.

Let the good times roll!

She placed the special needle for the chemo port, called a Huber needle, and injected saline to flush the catheter to make sure it wasn't blocked. She then hooked me up to my pump and began the pre-chemo treatment of Benadryl, Ativan, and anti-nausea medication. I didn't really pay attention to how long this took as I had decided that I was going to treat each chemo day as a day where I could sit back, relax, read or do anything I wanted – well at least within reach of my IV pole — without regard for time. My rules were I could binge watch Netflix, but only comedies; I could read, but only uplifting material, no death or tragedy; or I could work on the rug-hooking project I had brought, having all the materials I needed for what I came to call my chemo rugs. I figured I could start one (they are slow going for me) and see if I could get one done by the time chemo was complete in six months.

One of my dear friends had told me I was NOT to worry about dinners for the two nights after chemo, as she would be preparing them and bringing them to my house. I am famous for NOT asking ANYONE for help, **<u>EVER</u>**. Having someone care enough to do something like that had me feeling very vulnerable, but well-loved. It also had me feeling like it wouldn't be necessary as I was certain I was going to be one of those lucky ones for whom chemo would be a breeze.
I had no way of knowing at the time, but I would make several rugs as chemo made it difficult for me to concentrate on reading or plots and story lines; working with my hands seemed to be the easiest thing for me.

The pre-chemo drugs were all in my body and I was beginning to feel a little like my body was vibrating. Nothing unpleasant, but the way I feel when I take Benadryl. A lot of Benadryl. Less sleepy and more wired. Caffeinated without the jitters. A mild hum that radiated over my entire body.

Having gotten all the pre-chemo medications dripped into my body, it was now time to start the hard stuff. Nurse Angel Girl *told me that we would infuse my cocktails slowly this first time, just to see how my body would react. I was more of the attitude "let's get this shit over with as soon as possible," but that is not how it's done in the Oncology World.*

Drip. Drip. Drip.

Slowly the drugs began to drip into my body. Carboplatin would be first, Taxotere next, then Herceptin, followed lastly by Perjeta. It made no difference to me which went in when; they all had to go in, so just do it..

Every little bit Nurse Angel Girl would come over and ask me how I was feeling and if there was anything she could get or do for me. I felt pretty special with all the unnecessary attention. But for the most part I just sat back, watched ridiculous TV shows my kids had recommended, and let the drugs slowly drip into my body to do their magic and kill all those cancer cells — oh, and many healthy ones as well.

I had brought healthy snacks, but I didn't feel like eating. Not due to nausea or anything; more due to lack of activity. I'm usually a pretty busy person; sitting around in one place is unusual for me. I nibbled on some carrots and bleu cheese dressing and passed the time watching on my iPad and hooking my rug.

Drip, drip, drip.

Watching and hooking.

Hooking and watching something on my iPad, Nurse Angel Girl checked on me and commented that she was surprised I wasn't sound asleep with as much Benadryl as she had given me. I was pretty certain my thick hair was standing up on end for the exact same reason.

Then a little before noon my nose started to itch. Hmm, there must be something in the air in here. Every once in a while, I just had to rub my nose because it itched and it was also beginning to run. By chance, I happened to look up just as Nurse Angel Girl looked over the top of her computer at me in mid nose rub.

The itching continued.

[Didn't people receive the same packet I got that said not to wear perfume as some people are sensitive to it? Or maybe the rye grass was coming in. But so what, it was just an itchy nose!]

And the damn sitting for so long was starting to get to me. I was beginning to get a nagging ache in my lower back. I've had back issues for years, so I didn't see it as anything unusual, I just wish it had waited until later in the day. I decided to take a couple laps around the nurse's station and in to the TV room just to get up and about for a few minutes, and to stretch my legs and back.

Laps and stretching complete but still with an itchy nose and lower back ache, sliding back into my chair I could feel my ears begin to get warm and flush.

[Warm? How about hotter than the hinges of hell HOT!]

As I looked up after getting all settled in my recliner, stealthier than a ninja, Nurse Angel Girl was standing beside me.

She asked, "So what's going on."
Me, "Nothing. Why?"
"You feeling okay."
"Yeah, sure. Why?"
"I thought I saw your rubbing your nose."
"Well yeah. It itches."
"Ok. Anything else."

"Nope."

"Did I see you rubbing your back?"

"Well yeah, but it's just from sitting too long."

"Did you know your ears are really red?"

"Yeah, that happens to me. I have Ehler's Danlos and Mast Cell Activation Syndrome so I'm used to it."

"Actually, I think you are having a reaction to one of the drugs. I'm going to stop it for now and go talk to Dr. Medical Oncologist."

[WHAAAAT???]

Within moments a new person dropped by - the Pharmacist, who said, "I hear you are having a reaction to the Taxotere."

[What is this place that gossip travels so fast?]

"That's what Nurse Angel Girl said, but if this is as bad as it gets, this is really no big deal."

"Well, Nurse Angel Girl is speaking with Dr. Medical Oncologist and we will decide what to do next."

[Hey, sister, there's nothing to decide! Just keep giving me the damn medication. This is nothing.]

A few minutes later, Nurse Angel Girl came back and explained that Dr. Medical Oncologist wanted to stop the infusion for at least an hour; he wanted me to have additional steroids and Benadryl and then we would assess how I was in an hour.

In my mind, if Dr. Medical Oncologist didn't think these specific medications weren't important, he wouldn't have ordered them in the first place. I figured, unless my head started spinning around, I wasn't going to say another word about it. If he wanted me to have Taxotere, I was having

Taxotere. Little did I know, I didn't have to be such a stubborn tough gal.

About an hour later, with a slower infusion rate, we restarted the Taxotere. My nose itching diminished, my lower back didn't ache as much, and my ears, though still red, didn't feel like I needed ice to cool them off. The infusion dragged on, but eventually it was complete. Eight hours after walking through the front door, I had Chemo #1 behind me.

[Woo fucking hoo.]

Hubby picked me up. The Chef had left dinner the night before so, thankfully, I didn't have to think about that. Filled with steroids, enough Benadryl to subdue an elephant, Ativan for anxiety, and anti-nausea meds, plus with just the general unknown of what was ahead and with what felt like my hair still standing up straight on my head, I wasn't all that hungry, but at least my family wasn't going to starve. And I ate what I would later realize was my last normal meal for months.

Looking back at my journal, I noted I awoke the next morning feeling good, although I felt a tiny bit inexplicably odd: wired, body humming, and yet I could do my normal morning walk. I was to return to the oncology office for a Neulasta shot that afternoon; happy that I could at least drive myself to that. (Not being able to drive to or from Chemo was still pissing me off. I had heard so many people brag, "Why I drove myself to every single chemotherapy treatment." I felt as useless as the letter "G" in lasagna. Can't even drive to chemo. Sheesh. What a big baby!) Driving to the Neulasta shot at least made me feel a little better; not much but a little. Then a little later in the afternoon I began to feel a little queasy — kinda like morning sickness when I was pregnant, what my friend, The Cowgirl, called the urpies — plus, having been pretty regular most of my adult life, I was already feeling constipated.

[Well, I guess we now know which one would come first.]

The next couple days I spent trying to stay ahead of the nausea, sleeping poorly, and taking every medication they had given me for the constipation. If asked if I would rather be constipated or have diarrhea, I would pick diarrhea every time. But I managed to mow my lawn, worked out at the gym (even though it was slow going), and could do my usual work-related projects.

Day 4: I woke up. Well, more like I finally could not stand it anymore and got out of bed. I was sleeping poorly and the Neulasta shot had given me incredible bone and joint pain. I had severe growing pains as a child and this pain made those seem like an infantile introduction for the Neulasta side effects.

[And they said some people have no reaction at all to this shot!! Who are these people? I need to throat punch one!]

I was still trying to stay ahead of the nausea with the prescription medications, was taking Claritin and Aleve for the bone aches, but I had to get out of bed at 3 a.m. as I just couldn't stay there anymore. Now, besides the nausea and the bone pain, my mouth felt like I had swallowed the hottest coffee ever made and chased it down with a shooter of broken glass. And not just my mouth but down my throat, as well, so every time I swallowed my ears hurt, like I had strep throat.

[Well isn't this just a laugh a minute!]

Day 5 was a Monday — a typical gym day. I got there, but after just a few minutes of warming up, I suddenly started feeling like shit. My workout buddies and my trainer were the only ones that knew what was going on with me. I could see them watching me out of the corners of their eyes. And not just the corners; they were all keeping a really close eye on me. (The three of us had worked out together for two years, and so we were quite close and good friends.) My trainer could see me struggling and suggested I just stretch instead of working out. Stretching must have been good for me as I made it home just in time to have expulsive diarrhea.

[Guess we now know the order...constipation and then diarrhea.]

Great! Diarrhea, mouth sores, nausea, body aches, and now the scheduled appointment with the Gastroenterologist.

[Oh boy. Lucky me.]

The very first thing I did was apologize, "I'm sorry, but I'm just not feeling very well." Fortunately, I had my binder with me, as they had not received a copy of my PET scan. After reviewing the scan and conversing with me about the results of what looked to possibly be a spot of cancer on my colon, it was decided to do a colonoscopy as soon as possible. At that point I really didn't give a shit (actually I was giving plenty, scoping out a restroom everywhere I went). I just wanted the appointment over with. Everyone complains about how awful the prep for a colonoscopy is, so I figured, at this point, who cares. I already felt awful; how much worse could I possibly feel having to prep for a colonoscopy.

Lucky me! Dr. Poop Chute had an opening that Friday. Well...Dr. Medical Oncologist had said it shouldn't wait. I guess this was what not waiting looked like.

On my drive home, I stopped at the grocery store and purchased something I hadn't bought or eaten in two years. Crackers. Soda crackers and graham crackers. And bread. Thinking that I was going to be able to just go smoothly right along with my Paleo diet and life in general was now no longer a certainty. Crackers became my staple. With my mouth sores and nausea, crackers were about all I could tolerate. And now everything that crossed my lips tasted like I had been sucking on quarters all day.

[Yuuuummy!]

The next day was one-week post-chemo. I still felt awful but slept the best I had since the chemo treatment as the bone pain was beginning to subside a little each day. The best sleep was not great, but better than not at all. I hadn't walked or worked out for the past two days and was trying not to beat myself up for being such a wuss.

I was also trying to work. Through our construction company Hubby and I were working on a bid for a possible construction job, and I had things I was required to do in order for us to complete the bid. In cement shoes, I would drag into our office. Had I been the boss, I would have fired me for poor performance, or at least sent me home. Diarrhea, mouth sores, metallic taste in my mouth, body aches. And now I was running a low-grade fever. Good thing I needed to consume clear liquids to begin prepping for the colonoscopy because there wasn't much consuming of anything.

I felt like shit.

Thursday — just eight days past my first chemo — was blood draw day. I woke up feeling worse than I had felt so far and now every incision site, nick, scratch, and pimple were red and inflamed. My gut told me instinctively what was wrong, but one of the things I had PROMISED Hubby was that I was going to be a good cancer patient. I was going to follow ALL of the rules, which for me, included no self-diagnosing. I was totally giving myself over to my team. I hated it; but I had promised — both him and myself.

But I was still fairly certain I knew what was wrong.

I arrived at the office where the routine was that Nurse Angel Girl, or one of the other oncology nurses would draw my blood from my port. This facility has an on-site lab so as soon as they were done, I would see the doctor and he would review my labs. As she prepped her tray for the blood draw, she looked at me and said, "You don't look like you feel very well."

"I don't," I replied.

"What's wrong?"

[Was I on Candid Camera? What was wrong????? I have cancer for Christ's sake! I was eight days after my first chemo!!! What the hell do you think is wrong? Isn't this the way everyone feels during chemo?]

Fortunately, one of the other nurses interrupted our conversation as I'm not sure my response would have been in any way pleasant, even though I'm not sure I had the energy to say much of anything. But the gut feeling that I knew what was wrong would not go away. In my new role as good patient I was trying my hardest to just let them take care of me. (A note from future, wiser me: Being a good patient actually means speaking up about details. I know that now.) Quite honestly, since this was my first cycle, at this point, I assumed everybody must feel like this after chemo.

Yet, my gut was telling me it was more than just the chemo.

She finished her conversation and turned around to draw my blood. I unbuttoned my shirt to expose my port and the look on her face went from normal to very surprised in a split second. "Oh my!" she said.

"What's wrong?" I asked.

"Look at your port!"

I didn't need to.

I knew that along with every incision, nick, scratch, and pimple, my port site was also red, inflamed, and oozing. At that moment, it was actually the worst.

She continued, "I think your port is infected."

[Well, ain't that just fucking dandy! So much for my gut feeling.]

She now had to draw my blood from a vein in my arm, rather than my port.

[Good thing we paid for that expensive port!!]

This was a slow process as I was dehydrated. She then promptly took me back to see Dr. Medical Oncologist. When he entered the room, he said," I hear you aren't feeling well."

Me, "Nope."

At this point I was not a very good conversationalist, and my usual upbeat persona and wit were long gone. I wanted to have someone take me out back and just end my misery. My mouth and throat sores were worse, I ached EVERYWHERE, I was nauseated, there was no telling when I might have diarrhea, and all I wanted was to go home, lie on my couch, and never wake up again. I could feel tears beginning to well up in my eyes. I come from a long line of stoic, badass women, so crying is not something that happens frequently for me. That alone told me I was not in a very good place. Millions had done this before me and I was disappointed in myself for being such a big baby when I was certain I was pretty tough.

Dr. Medical Oncologist told me he was concerned it might be an infection in my port, that he wanted me to have some fluids, anti-nausea medications, and some antibiotics via IV while I was in his office. Once I was finished with the IVs, he then prescribed me oral antibiotics to take every day and told me he would see me for another blood draw the following week.

My gut still told me it wasn't an infected port. I was familiar with this feeling. Regardless, I had antibiotics, so I knew I had to be on my way to feeling better.

I realized, at this point, I was probably not going to be up for a colonoscopy, although I was certainly cleaned out. But I hadn't even thought about the prep; quite frankly I hadn't even thought about the colonoscopy in the past 48 hours. I cancelled the test and rescheduled it for the following Friday, knowing I would have to be feeling better by then.

The following day was Friday and I awoke feeling even worse yet. No longer was it a low-grade fever — it was a fever — and now I was vomiting. Once I could be up a bit and really look at my body, now every speck that had any inflammation was now a huge, hot, oozing wound. The incisions on my breast from the biopsies, the spots where the catheter of my port were tacked down, and now some new huge hot spots on one inner thigh, as well as a new one on my hip and an earlobe. Hot. Throbbing.

[Well, shit!]

Now I was certain what was wrong with me. This feeling was quite familiar.

I had strong antibiotics. Unfortunately, now everything I put in my body came back up or out. Antibiotics. Water. Pedialyte. Gatorade. Popsicles. In — quickly out from one end or the other.

[Oh look, a $50 pill floating in the toilet! I guess this is what they mean when they talk about flushing money away.]

Well if I wasn't going to be able to keep down water and antibiotics, how was I going to get better?

[FUUUUUCK!!]

And all the while I was trying to be brave in front of Hubby, not be a bother to him, AND do my part of the work proposal. We were stressed with the bid due that afternoon and I certainly didn't want to add to that stress, but in my current shape, I wasn't really much of a help.

I tried to act normal (as normal as a vomiting, shit-storm cancer patient can act) and I quietly called Dr. Medical Oncologist's office and told them I wasn't feeling any better and couldn't keep down the antibiotics. They told me to come in as soon as I could get there.

Suddenly, I realized I was going to have to do something that I find extremely hard to do.

I was going to have to ask for help.

[Noooooo!!!]

I would rather walk through broken glass than ask for help; but Hubby was now trying to finish our big proposal and I was, now, no longer able to assist him. There was no way possible he was going to be able to drop everything and take me to the doctor's office, my daughter was in New York, my son was at school, and my mom was no longer driving. I was actually aware enough (and actually listened to that awareness) that I knew I was not in any condition to drive myself to the doctor.

Furthermore, I knew I needed to resolve this SOON, as it was Friday. The weekend was going to be here in the blink of an eye and I was declining rapidly.

168

I knew I needed to call someone, and I knew exactly who it was. But when you are used to doing pretty much everything yourself, for me, it was one of the hardest calls I've ever had to make.

So, I negotiated with myself. If I threw up one more time I would call. Then I would have to renegotiate the parameters, as that first one failed.

If I had another episode of expulsive diarrhea, then I'd call.

Okay, if I threw up ANOTHER time AND had diarrhea, then I would call.

As sick as I was, the negotiations with myself lasted about 30 minutes or maybe even longer. I even began to look up taxi cab numbers just so I wouldn't have to bother anyone. But when I pinched the skin on the top of my hand and it just stayed that way, I knew I needed to get to the doctor. I was vomiting, had diarrhea, a temperature of 103 degrees, I ached all over, and every little spot on my body throbbed like when you hit your thumb with a hammer.

Then I started to cry. Now I knew I was REALLY sick.

I shut myself in the bathroom and curled up on the floor in fetal position and between vomiting and diarrhea, I cried. This was not going at all like I planned. The having no problems. Breezing right through chemotherapy. Life as usual. None of this was happening. Dammit!! Didn't this cancer know who I am. I am Ann Fucking Low, DAMMIT!! I'm badass.

But cancer didn't give a shit.

This was fucked.

FUCKED. FUCKED. FUCKED!

After about 10 minutes I wobbled my way to the couch and my phone and dialed my friend, Mama Bear.

I practiced in my head what I was going to say and, with a sore mouth and throat, no energy, and no idea when my next hurl/expel session might occur, I dialed her number. Secretly I hoped she wouldn't answer and then I could just stay on my couch and wait to either get better or die. At that moment I was hoping for dying.

As I expected, she answered right away.

[SHIT!]

I was trying to sound casual and nonchalant, "Hey. Sorry to bother you, but I was wondering if you were doing anything right now. And it's totally okay if you are in the middle of something."

She replied, "No I'm good. What's up?"

"I'm not feeling very well, and the doctor wants to me to come into the office. Unfortunately, Hubby is working on a bid that is due this afternoon and he can't take me. Would it be a terrible inconvenience to run me to my doctor's office and drop me off? It's okay if you can't."

My house is probably, driving safely and conservatively, 15 minutes away from hers. She was ringing my doorbell 10 minutes later. Her "Oh honey!" when she first saw me told me all I needed to know. I must have looked as bad as I felt.

First, I apologized for having to call her.

Then I apologized because I was going to need to carry an emesis basin, those cute little kidney-bean-shaped plastic bowls they give you to vomit into at the hospital. (I always called them my nemesis basin as there are few things I hate more than puking.)

We arrived at the office and I asked her to just drop me off; I would be fine. Nope. Not Mama Bear. She got me inside and then she took over. In the shape I was in, that was exactly what I needed. As the wife of a physician, she knows the medical game. As someone who saw me fall and break my arm without ever shedding a tear, she knew I was in bad shape when I started to cry as soon as I saw Nurse Angel Girl.

Angel Girl asked me what was going on, and between breaks for me to puke, I was able to communicate how I was feeling and what was going on. And for the first time I broke my promise to be what I thought was a good patient and told her what my gut was telling me was wrong.

"I think I have a staph infection."

There. I had said it out loud. The pesky bastard that had made my life miserable a couple years before and had been rattling around in my mushy brain for the past few days, had passed over my lips, and was now right there in the infusion room like a big pink elephant. There he was, Mr. Staph Infection.

With my concern having been brought to life just by having spoken it, within minutes of my arrival, I was again being infused with fluids, antibiotics, and anti-nausea medication. With little relief from the diarrhea and vomiting, everything else seemed to be getting worse as well. The body aches and pains were now almost intolerable. New inflamed, aching spots showed up in additional locations as the day grew longer. BIG. THROBBING. HOT. SORE. OOZING.

Infusion personnel came by. "This is NOT how chemo is supposed to go," to which I replied, "I think I have a staph infection."

The Pharmacist came by, "We are on the phone with your insurance company to try to find out the strongest antibiotic we can put you on that they will pay at least a portion of."

I responded, "I think I have a staph infection."

The Nurse Practitioner breezed over, "I think I have a staph infection."

Other oncology nurses, checking on me and changing out my IV bags, "I think I have a staph infection." Someone was always checking on me, so I knew I was in good hands, but I felt like they were still all sure my port was the problem. And I was pretty sure I had a staph infection. I was way past being the good patient and now I was the patient who was telling everyone what I thought was wrong.

Even though I tried and tried to send her home, Mama Bear did not leave my side the entire day. She gave me tissues when I cried. She hovered. She talked to her own hubby, a physician, to get his opinion. She intervened when someone would come over if I was lucky enough to fall asleep for a few moments. She covered me with blankets when I had chills and gave me water when I was burning up. She took over and, for one of the first times in my adult life, I let someone do that. I had never felt more exposed and vulnerable in my life. I let go of the needing to be in control, to be the strong one, and let her take over. She was a lifesaver on that day; and to this day I would do anything for her.

But I started to get concerned as 4 o'clock neared.

4 o'clock. ON A FRIDAY!

No definitive answers from my insurance company.

No plan yet.

And I still felt like shit.

Things were not looking too good.

Finally, the Pharmacist and Dr. Medical Oncologist came over to tell me that they had finally heard from my insurance company. The antibiotics they would like to send me home with were $4000. Four. Thousand. Dollars.

[You have got to be FUCKING kidding me??!!!!]

I just shook my head. If I wasn't nauseated already, I certainly would have been after hearing that little bit of news. Not only was it going to be impossible financially, it made no sense to me to take oral antibiotics, given I was not having much success keeping anything down. At $4000 this was going to be some even more expensive vomit than the previous batch. I told them that plan was NOT an option.

With the sands of the hourglass quickly filling the bottom and with the top almost empty, they tried to get several other options authorized by my insurance company.

Home health care — Nope.

Different antibiotics — Nope.

Finally, I looked at Dr. Medical Oncologist and asked, "Why don't you just admit me?"

Dr. Medical Oncologist replied, "We just don't normally admit patients."

I said, "Double check with my insurance, but I think once I'm admitted as an emergency, everything will be covered."

About 20 minutes later I saw the Pharmacist, Dr. Medical Oncologist, and Nurse Angel Girl walking my way like a sheriff and his posse. The plan was in place. They had called my insurance and called the hospital. I was going to be admitted for "Cellulitis".

I did not give a shit what the diagnosis was, and I never thought I would say this...EVER...but I was happy to be going to the hospital. As happy as someone who has been puking for hours can be. It was 5:20 on a Friday afternoon and knowing I was going someplace where help was just the push of a button away was such a relief. I just wanted to get there and curl up in a ball and be taken care of. I was past being badass. There wasn't an ounce of strong left in me. I was sick, and I actually wanted to be where they take care of sick people.

The only disappointment was that Mama Bear couldn't take me directly to the hospital, as there were no beds yet available. The plan was for her to take me home and Hubby would take me to the hospital when we were called that the bed was available.

Fortunately, that was not long at all — only about 15 minutes after arriving home. Unfortunately, off the IV anti-nausea drugs and fluids, the vomiting quickly returned, and I was now quickly going backwards again. By the time we were at the hospital, I was back to using my "nemesis" basin and was ready to just be taken out back and put out of my misery again. There wasn't one ounce of spunk left in me.

At this hospital, they collect all your insurance documentation, medical history, and officially admit you while you are already in your room. My admission took place with the Admissions Counselor standing outside the bathroom door asking me questions between my praying to the porcelain god and pleading to die. Not until they had all that information could they start treating me.

Fortunately, prior to starting treatment, I had put all my medications on a note in my cell phone. Then at Dr. Medical Oncologist's I had made notes of the various medications and antibiotics I had been given throughout the day. When I was asked by my admitting nurse if I knew what medications I had been given that day I could rattle all of them off with dosage and time as if they were my children's birthdates. Although she took it in stride, Hubby was impressed. At least I could still make an impression on someone!

Once I was sitting on my bed instead of kneeling over the toilet, I sent Hubby home. Again, what was he going to do for me by staying? Listen to me puke? Watch the new sores pop up on my neck and face? Start the IV? (They were still working from the premise that my port was infected so they did not want to enter the port.) I felt better having him home keeping our little boat afloat, which now included letting the kids and our parents know I was in the hospital.

From my special room reserved for patients either having hematology issues or patients receiving chemotherapy, over the course of the next several hours I met an entirely new group of caregivers. More oncology nurses. Hospitalists. A social worker. Nurse's aides. Rest was not in the game plan with the constant blood draws, checks of my vital signs, and reviews of how my symptoms were doing. And of course, the continued vomiting and diarrhea. However, I was grateful to be where I could get pain medications, anti-nausea medicines, and fluids. I wasn't feeling much better yet, but I knew within a few hours there, I would have to start!

An even better feeling for me was that Hubby was free of having to take care of me. He is supportive in every way, but when it comes to medical stuff, he is way out of his league. I'm not sure who was more relieved I was in the hospital, me, or him.

During my day in Dr. Oncologist's office, I had checked in on Mom. Her cold had not gotten any better, and she seemed worse. I recall that I texted my brother that Mom was not feeling better, that I was at the hospital, so could he check on her. And I could have hallucinated all that (except the part about Mom being sick) given I was delirious most of that day. The following morning, my first morning in the hospital, I called Mom to check on her. I immediately knew she was not doing well. I don't recall if I contacted my brother to check on her, or if she did, or how it occurred (to this day some things still remain blurry about that time) but soon my brother was strolling into my room, as he had brought Mom to the emergency room. I knew that I must be starting to feel a little bit better because I found that incredibly funny. Mom and daughter, both in the same hospital. My worry about her replaced any concern I had for myself.

At some point the previous night they had taken a sample of one of my oozing sores. In the early afternoon, a familiar face walked into my room – Dr. Infectious Disease."

I chuckled when we simultaneously said, "Hey, I recognize you!" (I must have been feeling a little better — I could actually chuckle!) There before me stood the infectious disease doctor who had treated my original staph infection after I broke my ankle two years prior.

He let me know that I, again, had a staph infection and that we would be monitoring my white blood cell counts to see if I was going to have to follow the regimen I had previously with my ankle, which was 42 days of IV antibiotics three times a day. To add to my fun, my fourth IV had failed, and I was waiting for the team that were going to put in a PICC line. A PICC line is a Peripherally Inserted Central Catheter. Fancy lingo for an IV that is typically in the upper arm and advanced until the catheter tip ends in a large vein in the chest, near the heart. My port was still considered off limits, my IV's had failed multiple *times, so a PICC line only made sense given there was no conversation about me busting out of the hospital any time soon. While waiting for the nurses who would place my PICC line, my brother returned to tell me they were going to be admitting Mom for pneumonia. I apologized that he had to take over, as I'm the one that is usually the caregiver in these situations, but I assured him I would be well in no time and would be able to take her home.*

The good news for me was that, slowly, I was starting to feel better.

Later, I had one of the nurses check to see where Mom was. Not only were we in the same hospital, but she was in a room on the same floor! When I could convince one of the nurses to get me a rolling IV pole, and with the admonishment that if I spent more than two minutes in Mom's room they were going to come get me and I wouldn't be allowed to leave my room again, I shuffled down to check on her.

With Mom in the good hands of her pulmonologist, me in the incredibly capable hands of my team, and with my colonoscopy rescheduled, I could concentrate on getting better. There really wasn't much to concentrate on. Mainly I was just sitting around waiting to feel better. My family and a few friends came to visit, (I hadn't told anyone I was in the hospital, but news travels fast anyway) and each day I felt a little better. I knew I was advancing down the road to recovery as I now wanted to go home. I was tired of the hospital.

After four days, Dr. Infectious Disease delivered news that was sweet nectar to my waxy ears. I was stable enough that I could bust outta that joint and be on oral antibiotics for the next several weeks rather than through a PICC line.
I had turned the corner.

I was very shaky, but given that in just a short 50 days I had gone from working out like a fiend or hiking every day, to having been told I had cancer, had two biopsies, two MRIs, a PET scan, a port placement, a chemotherapy session, and had just spent five days in the hospital. Shaky seemed expected, at this point.

Weak and wobbly, but glad to be home, little by little I began to feel better. Then, I noticed my scalp began to feel odd. Itchy, but not really. Prickly, but more just a sensation of a slight tingle; kind of like when your hair blows the wrong way, or how it feels right after you take it out of a ponytail. Like you just want to rub your fingers all over your scalp. It was when I started to feel these sensations, and would run my fingers through my hair, that my hair began to come out. First just a few strands. Then tufts. Clumps followed. On my brush. On my clothes. In my purse. All over the floor. On my pillow and in the bed.

I guess somehow, I thought I would feel some sort of sensation when it started coming out, but it just came out. Everywhere! There would be no committing the perfect crime right now. I was leaving DNA everywhere I went.

I tolerated that trail of hair loss for less than 12 hours. After John left for school and Hubby was off to work, I went in search of our electric clippers.

While searching for the clippers I received a text from Mama Bear that a mutual friend of ours had passed away from her cancer fight. I know I was shaky from my medications and all I had just gone through, but the news of her passing was another severe kick in the ovaries. A HARD one. I sat in a chair and let the news wash over me. I felt horrible for her family. The more I thought about it, the harder the news seemed. We were acquaintances, but the news felt devastating. I sat in silence trying to figure out why it seemed so disturbing.

And then it struck me. For the first time, I thought — that could be me. That could be MY family having to deal with that loss. It broke my heart.

With the news of the death of our friend fresh on my mind, I shaved my head as best as I could by myself. Now sporting a buzz cut that I suspected looked like it had been done by a four-year-old, with oozing, but healing, sores all over my face, neck, and other parts of my body, when I finally got a chance to look in the mirror, I totally lost it.

Looking much like a war refugee and feeling like shit, mentally and physically, I reached out to one of the people I consider my biggest supporter, my daughter, Landry.

I texted her to see if she was free to Skype. As soon as I saw her face, all I could do was sob. That hadn't been my intention, but as soon as I saw her beautiful face, I could no longer hold it together. I was pretty fragile physically, and mentally I was not all that great either. I told her what had been going on and how awful I felt — which was sick, sore, and dreadful. She's an incredibly amazing young woman. (I would like her even if she wasn't mine!) She listened. But when I told her how ugly I looked and felt, she said exactly what I needed to hear.

She asked, "Mom. Don't you always tell me I'm a mini-you?"
"Yes," I blubbered, with bubbles of snot coming out my nose.

"Then how do you think it makes me feel when you say something like that to me?" she asked.
Like I said, she knew exactly what to say to me. I had lost sight that this wasn't just about me. We were all being affected by this.

I took a deep breath.

I actually took several and I chose to snap out of it.

179

Talking with her got me back to where I could remember that things work out best for those who make the best of how things work out. It was time for me to find my sense of humor again and make the best of the situation.

John was the first to come home. We have a large property with two homes; we live in one and he was living in the other. And he made it a habit of saying goodbye every morning and would check on me every evening as soon as he arrived home from school or work. He walked into the house and around the corner, "Hi, Mo......oh, Mom! Your hair!"

It wasn't negative or positive. It was almost like, for the first time, it finally got real for him. I'm not sure if that is the case or not, but the tone, the way he said it, and the expression on his face went straight through my heart. Not because I was sick, but for him having a sick mom. To me there was a huge difference. I hated for my kids to have a sick mom. It broke my heart.

*Later he was willing to use the clippers and clean up the worst haircut ever and suggest that I should go to a professional and have it cleaned up even a little better. I laughed. I assured him that I was pretty certain that it would not be necessary. At the rate my hair was coming out, I would be bald in no time.
I was right.*

As I look back over my notes of that period of time, I see I broke Mom out of the hospital a couple of days after I got out and later in the week saw Dr. Medical Oncologist, where he told me we needed to postpone the colonoscopy until after I was done with chemotherapy. He did not want to risk any additional stress or potential infections possibly being introduced into my body at that time.

And each day I wrote that I started to feel better and better until on Sept. 30 I jotted: Best day so far! Feel almost normal!

Too bad the next day was CHEMO DAY!

Again, John drove me to chemo and he tried to walk me in. I assured him I was fine, hugged him, and watched him drive away. I then promptly turned around and puked in the garbage can located several feet away from the outside entrance.

Embarrassed, I was assured that it was not uncommon for that to occur. Pre-treatment anxiety. Another cancer surprise! For me it wasn't the anxiety of the day of chemo, but apprehension of what the next couple of weeks would be like. Cycle one had not gone easily. I was nervous about cycle two.

Pre-treatment anxiety was something that I never got over. It occurred every cycle. John would drop me off — I would stand outside until he drove away — then I would puke in the parking lot.

Pre-chemo went pretty much the same as the first cycle; the drugs were started and soon it would be time for the Taxotere. Not long after starting it, my nose started to itch and my lower back began to ache. Nurse Angel Girl noticed immediately and stopped the infusion. Apparently Taxotere was not going to be my friend. Lost in the hub-bub of the staph infection was that somewhere in there Dr. Medical Oncologist had told me that if I had a reaction to the Taxotere again, we would need to change the medication to one of Taxotere's sister drugs. I felt that, if Taxotere was his first choice, that was the medication I wanted to have. However, when Nurse Angel Girl shared that the next side effect of Taxotere — after the itching, aches, and flushing — was asphyxiation, I agreed it probably was best that we change it. I finished the rest of my chemo with Abraxene, with none of the infusion side effects of the Taxotere.

Cancer can be a moving target.

Lucky me, my birthday was five days later; right about the time when I would start feeling my worst. Hubby asked me, "What do you want to do for your birthday?"

John asked me, "What do you want to do for your birthday, Mom?"

My response to both was the same — absolutely nothing.

From New York, Landry had told me she wanted to throw me a "surprise" party. You would have to know me to know that I DO NOT LIKE SURPRISES. I like throwing surprises; I just hate getting surprised. When she brought it up, I was begging her, "Please, please, please, don't do this." Her response was, "Don't worry, Mom. You will love it."

[Oh, HELL no!]

She requested the contact information of all the people who were watching over me and checking on me and for the friends that she didn't have contact information for. After many days of my not sending it — thinking if I just ignored it, she would get too busy and forget — she browbeat me into creating a list and emailing it to her. I felt nauseated at the prospect of whatever she was planning. I kept asking her to tell me what it was, but all she would tell me was, "Don't worry, Mom. You will love it."

[NO, I WON'T!]

She knew me well enough to know I would HATE a party. I HATE being the center of attention and I was upset that she insisted on going ahead with it, knowing I wouldn't like it.

I was sitting with Hubby and whining about the fact that she had something planned when I heard the garage door opening. This was not unusual as John was due home from school and work and often came in this way to check on me. But it was completely unusual when he walked through the door with Landry trailing him. I was over the moon with excitement. It was the best surprise ever!!

She had decided that she needed to come home and see me as the rest of her school year was going to be too intense for many visits. She decided, at the last minute, to buy a ticket, hop on a plane, and come home and surprise me.

I was so thrilled!

But the next day it struck me that there was still a "surprise" party to worry about. And now with her home it was even MORE worrisome. But she didn't mention it, so I was optimistic that her coming home was the surprise, she had gotten too busy at school or had realized that to arrange something like that from New York was just too difficult and it wasn't going to happen.

[A girl can dream, can't she?]

This cycle of chemo was pretty much following the same pattern as the first, but gratefully without the staph infection. Between constipation and diarrhea, vomiting, and bone pain, if there WAS going to be a surprise party, I was going to be the worst Birthday Girl ever. I was just happy to have my little family together, even if it was just for a few days.

I'm not sure why, but for some reason I wanted to do something we had never done with the kids and go to Benihana's for dinner on the night of my birthday. Quite honestly, I was already at the feel crappy phase, but I put a smile on my face and pretended all was fine. A little while before it was time for me to get ready, John took me next door to his house as he insisted he needed to show me something.

[Can't this wait?]

When we came back in to the house THERE WAS MY SURPRISE PARTY! Our friend Weezer was there and all over the table were cards and gifts. Piles of them. Landry HAD arranged a surprise party. Here is what she emailed to the "invitees:"

Hello!

Since I can't be home for my beautiful, wonderful mother's birthday (on Monday, October 6th) , I wanted to plan her a surprise party.

However, as I'm sure you know, with her health the way it is, I don't think she would be super psyched to be flocked by a huge group of people without her consent.

So instead of surprising her with your presence, I was hoping I could convince you to write her a letter instead. The best part of a letter is that it's a tangible form of support that she can go back and read/revisit anytime she needs to.
I know she always struggles asking for help and this is a way that she can access the support she needs, whenever she needs it, without even having to ask.

Actual gifts are definitely not necessary, but if that's something you're interested in, I know she's been seeking out cool scarves/hats/etc that won't make her look completely ridiculous (as most of the scarves and such designed for the purposes she needs them for are totally weird and lame). Of course, if there is anything else that you may have in mind, go for it, but again, gifts are not necessary.

I have enlisted the help of my dad and brother (I cc'd them in on this email) to coordinate the actual delivery of the goods. The idea is to have all of the letters and such together (my dad will take her out to eat or something while my brother sets everything up in a party fashion) so that it's like a surprise party, without having to be overwhelmed by a bunch of people.

There are a few options for delivery:

1. If you are out of town/far away/etc. — you can send it to:
Chris Low
XXXXX X XXXXX
Phoenix, Az 85028

If this is the best way for you, PLEASE makes sure you send it within the next day or so in order to make sure they get it in time

2. You can potentially drop it off/leave it with my brother or dad. This, however, will require a little bit of coordination as, of course, you'd need to do so at a time or place when/where my mother won't be around.
Their phone numbers are:
xxx-xxx-xxx (Chris)
xxx-xxx-xxx (John)

3. My brother has also offered to pick up letters/etc on Sunday and Monday if the first two options don't work for you. Just send him a text/call at xxx-xxx-xxxx.

Feel free to email, call, or text me with any questions! My number is xxx-xxx-xxx.

Thank you for all of the love and support you have given my mom.

Not only does it mean the world to her, but to me as well — especially since I am so far away.

I cannot express my gratitude enough and I so look forward to hearing from her on Monday as to how it all goes!

Thanks again,
Landry

And they had all been involved. John and Hubby picking up letters and cards and gifts without me having any idea. It was the most amazing, thoughtful, gift she could have arranged. For someone who prides herself on not crying, I was having a hard time not weeping with the touching sentiments that people had shared in their letters to me. I was so moved and touched. It was awesome. Definitely my kind of surprise party! Like Landry had said, "You will love it."

And I did! And with her deciding to hop a flight and be there as well — for a short time — all was right in my world.

We went to dinner, and although I was feeling horrible, I didn't want them to know. And I was getting sad that, as soon as we were done with dinner, we had to take Landry to the airport. I have always kidded that, if I knew my kids were going to leave me, I would have never had the brats, but I think when you are going through a critical illness, that is even more the sentiment. Putting her back on a plane was ripping my heart out.

After the meal, we drove to the house and while they were gathering Landry's things, without the rest of my family knowing, I was losing my dinner. Bye, bye Benihana's birthday dinner!

We took Landry to the airport. Then it was back to cancer as usual.

I had been told that each cycle was usually the same as the previous but over time there might be a cumulative effect, so cycle 5 and 6 would probably be my hardest. That was pretty accurate as my three weeks usually went like this: four to five days of constipation, three to four days of diarrhea, bone pain for five days, two weeks of feeling pretty nauseated and/or vomiting, blood work every week, and then feeling better just in time for John to drop me off, for me to puke in the outside garbage can, and to do it all over again.

Chemotherapy is a funny thing in how differently it affects everyone. It was definitely not something I knew before. I thought everyone who got the same drugs would have similar side effects. But as our bodies are all individual, so is the reaction to chemotherapy.

Even though I had, usually, two weeks that I felt pretty horrible, I still attempted to walk every day. No longer able to go to the gym, I was moving slower than I had the previous month, but at least I was still moving. Moving and occasionally puking in bushes in my neighborhood.

All through my chemo I tried to do ONE big thing each day. Some days it was just a load of laundry. Toward the end of a cycle, when I might be feeling a little better, it could be mowing the lawn. Regardless, I was beginning to realize that no matter how badass and tough I thought I was, I was most definitely not on my "A" game. And other days I needed to be on injured reserves, as chemo was plain kicking my ass!!

Chemotherapy eventually ended, although I would still have another six months of Herceptin, so there was no big celebration and I didn't have to tell Nurse Angel Girl goodbye just yet. Other than the staph infection challenge setting me back physically, through most of chemo I still did many of the things I always did: work, yard work, walking, and hiking. I probably could have gone to the gym but fast movements nauseated me and I didn't think my trainer would have gone easy on me. He trains Navy SEALs. And I'm the kind of girl who, when he challenged me to do something, would go, "Oh yeah! WATCH THIS!" I didn't think that was probably the best for me through this. So, for once I listened to my body, my practical self and I stuck to walking and hiking.

After my last treatment, I met with Dr. Medical Oncologist, who said the time had come to go visit Dr. Breast Surgeon. I needed to be off chemo for three weeks and then he was recommending that we proceed with my surgery.

The three weeks flew by and I was back in my breast friend's care in what seemed a blink of an eye. Dr. Breast Surgeon again reviewed our options. After waffling and wavering and deciding and then changing my mind multiple times, I elected to have a double mastectomy with reconstruction. He honored my decision without a bat of an eye, which I really appreciated, as I was fearful that I was going to get a lecture about conserving the healthy breast. I had struggled for months to make my decision; I just wasn't up for any more conversation trying to change my mind. Fortunately, his response was, "Okay" and we just moved on to the specifics. I reminded him about the staph infection and after acknowledging that we would aggressively treat it, he explained his part of the surgery, what he would do with the breast tissue, my pesky little lymph nodes, and that I would stay overnight in the hospital, perhaps two if necessary.

One of the things he shared was that since I was having reconstruction, we could actually schedule the surgery so that Dr. Plastic Surgeon could be there at the same time. This way Dr. Plastic Surgeon could place the expanders during the mastectomies, thus cutting out an additional separate surgery, as the goal was to get me on to radiation in eight weeks. I was all for combining surgeries.

[Let's do this!]

January 19 - my mother's birthday - became the "free the girls" date.

Back at Dr. Plastic Surgeon's office, we let the girls out to play for one of the last times, certainly the last time that THESE girls would be free in his office. He covered the surgical process, the placement of the expanders, the fact that they would be slightly expanded at surgery, and that I would have drains for seven to 10 days. Once the drains were removed, he would begin to fill the expanders until we got to the size I wanted (a nice perky B sounded good to me!) and then I would be ready for radiation. We wanted to complete the implant exchange before radiation as the success rate of plastic surgery drops dramatically in a radiated breast, due to the changes in the skin, both externally and internally. He explained the bandages that would be covering my empty boob bags and showering rules and gave me the restrictions on activity, and with a last reminder of my staph infection, I took my bald badass-self off and began to prepare for the following Monday's double mastectomy.

I prepared by writing and here's part of what I shared on my blog:

<u>The Big Day!</u>

As I've grown older, I have come to realized that sometimes we have friends that with time we no longer have a positive relationship with, or we have such big differences that we need to cut them entirely out of our lives for our own sanity and health. Today, that day has come for me.

This is the day I remove a couple of girls – close friends – from my life – forever!

With these two, who have been around since the summer I turned 11, it often seems like they have caused me more problems in this long relationship than they have been worth. From the moment they showed up, they became the center of attention. They were always first in the room without a need to announce their arrival. Just their mere presence was enough to attract notice, stares and even more often some kind of comment. Over the years there has been me…. the introvert, standing back watching….and my two obvious and obnoxious friends creating mayhem in their paths, and letting everyone know when a room was cold.

I've spent 40 years in a very strange relationship with these two. I have wished they were different. I have worked out so hard and ridden my bicycle literally THOUSANDS of miles hoping they couldn't keep up and would just fade away. But they have always just hung in there.

But today is the day I cut these two girls out of my life forever. Today is the day of my double mastectomy – a decision I did not come to easily. And even with all the things they tell me that can go wrong – infections, rejection, leaking, scarring that can lead to an unusual shape and all the other complications – even including a recurrence – I KNOW I'm making the right decision for all of us. But it didn't come easily and I'm glad I've had the past few months of chemotherapy to think about it; time to ask other survivors what they did and how they feel about the procedure and the results – time to process the information and to come to terms with whatever my decision was going to be.

So here we are – just a few bittersweet hours before removing from my life both of these girls that have been with me for the past 40 years; the two most obvious things about my body…and although I'm feeling very anxious and nervous, I am very comfortable with my decision to say good bye to these two….these two trouble makers and life givers.

Regardless of what our relationship has been – you will be missed!

Bon Voyage Breasticles Day arrived way too quickly. Hubby dropped me off with the promise to see me later in the day. With my fuzzy chemo brain at its worst, there is actually very little of those two days that I truly remember. I remember checking in. I remember being in the pre-op area wearing the awesome beanie my daughter had given me. (I put the surgical cap over it, so I could keep wearing it. I suspect they removed it once I was in medical LaLa land rather than the chemo LaLa land I was living in then.) I recall the nurse teaching me how to empty the drains and record my progress. If Dr. Breast Surgeon or my family came to visit, I have no recollection of it. I remember getting in the car at the hospital when Hubby came to pick me up. I remember getting a smoothie on the way home, but I don't remember much until the following day.

Our body is an amazing machine. If you remove an organ from the body, you create a big empty space that naturally fills with fluid as the body responds to the missing tissue. The body will eventually adjust to the missing tissue and produce less fluid to fill that space, so the drains that are put there to reduce the buildup of fluids (seroma) then can be removed.

Or that's usually the how it works.

The next few days were really just a blur of taking it pretty easy, emptying the drains, logging my progress, and counting the days until I was producing less the 20 cc's of fluid each day and could get those little plastic grenades removed from my body, in the seven to 10 days that was the usual rate of recovery.

At one week, on the first visit back with Dr. Plastic Surgeon, I was still producing much more fluid than I expected to be at seven days. Dr. Plastic Surgeon didn't seem too concerned, as he shared that often the serous (fluid) production abruptly stops. I was to come in to the office if that happened before our next visit, which was scheduled for a week away.

[A week away?!]

I knew I would be seeing him way before a week was out. I needed to get the drains pulled so we could finish the reconstruction before I had radiation, as Dr. Plastic Surgeon shared that the success rate of reconstruction dropped dramatically if completed after radiation. So, it was important (No! Imperative!) to get the drains out soon to exchange the expanders for implants and then move on to radiation.

But another seven days passed with me walking the 57 steps back and forth to my workshop, working, and still taking it pretty easy. I also had a Herceptin infusion and a blood draw, and every day I emptied the drains that had now become these little bulbs of frustration.

[Dammit! Stop filling up!]

No change. I was still producing as much fluid as day 1.
Another visit with Dr. Plastic Surgeon arrived, and again he reassured me that one day I may wake up and things would be

different. As soon as I produced 20 cc's or less, I was to get to his office and he would immediately remove the drains.

Empty. Measure. Record.
[COME ON!]

Empty. Measure. Record.
[Are you kidding me?]

Empty. Measure. Record.
[What. The. Fuck!!!!]

Empty. Measure. Record.
[God dammit.]

Empty. Measure. Record.
[You have got to be fucking kidding me!!!]

And then it started happening. [Insert music. Nope – not that happy upbeat kind. That dramatic – something bad is going to happen music.] I woke up and I could tell something had changed.

Empty. Measure. Record.
[SHIT!]

Empty, measure, record, take my temperature.
[REALLY?????! Can't a girl catch a break here!]

The digital thermometer was not kind to me. The oral mercury thermometer confirmed it. I was sick.

So, 20 days beyond the seven to 10-day limit for having the now-loathsome plastic grenades in my body, my temperature was at 102 degrees and I was feeling like I had just been to Fight Club. I headed off to Dr. Plastic Surgeon's office for an unscheduled visit.

He confirmed what I already knew: I had ANOTHER staph infection. What I didn't know, until that moment, was that he would need to pull the drains.

[WHAAAATT???Aren't I still producing a bunch of fluid in those shitty little plastic things?]

Here I was, again, in a situation where I had NO control of anything in this process. I was incredibly mentally deflated.

But physically I would be inflated very soon. Unfortunately, with no drains in place, where my breasts used to be — my boob bags — quickly filled, and I suddenly had big breasticles again.

[You bitches! You try to kill me and even though you've been lopped off you are still going to be causing problems. Fuck you both! Fuck chemo! Fuck reconstruction! Fuck cancer!]

This was one of the lowest points in my treatment. I was so depressed and felt so awful that for the very first time I wished I had done nothing. No mammogram. I wished the original radiologist had missed the teeny-weeny spot. No chemo. And certainly, no surgery. I was so over all of it.

I still had all the faith in Dr.'s Plastic Surgeon and Breast Surgeon, but I sure knew there must be something wrong with ME.

And I was still so over it.

My core support squad kept in touch and I shared what was physically going on, but I intentionally did not share where I was mentally. Jane Wayne is ingrained in my DNA and, my core reasoning went, I didn't want anyone to worry about me when they all had their own stuff to deal with. Quite frankly, I was afraid if I told anyone, including my family, just how fragile my mental state was at that moment that the little tiny thread of sanity I was hanging on to with bone-white knuckles would fray more and finally snap and I would be receiving the rest of my care in a mental ward.

Looking back, I can admit it was very lonely and not one of my smartest decisions. I felt I was all alone and the medication I had been taking for anxiety might as well have been a breath mint. My anxiety had me fully in its grasp. I was sick, afraid, felt all alone and I was questioning all my medical decisions up to that point. Maybe those recommended coffee enemas to cure cancer would have been the better answer. Maybe. What if. Could have. And I was "shoulding" all over myself.

Isolation Nation was now my home.

I was no longer able to take my daily walks or hikes; so I took the 57 steps to our workshop and 57 back. Took the antibiotics. Watched the girls grow. Pretended to be ok. I was deep in a black hole that that I was sure I would never dig my way out. It never occurred to me to ask for help from my trusted team of medical pros, loving family, and reliable friends. But having seen so many others on social media breeze through their treatment, I felt like a pathetic loser.

On the bright side, with my boob bags full of fluid, I had a preview of what the girls were going to look like as a perky "B" rather than a saggy "D".

Even through all of this, I was still taking FIL and Mom to doctor appointments. I was still getting Herceptin. And all the while I would just slap a smile on my face and put one foot in front of the other. I really didn't know what else to do besides that. This was completely new territory and was out of my control. I was on the rollercoaster ride and stubbornly choosing to ride alone. At this point I could no longer put my hands over my head, even if I wanted to. There was nothing enjoyable about where I was, and I felt too awful to even hold on. I was just on the rollercoaster and not even sure if I was strapped in — I was just on the ride.

And it sucked!

Back at Dr. Plastic Surgeon's office, I was pretending to be fine with the process. He told me that he felt the infection was under control. He felt that the seromas were too big to absorb on their own and that we needed to surgically put the drains back in.

[SERIOUSLY??!! This fun just never ends!]

With the drains surgically placed back where they had been, time stood still. I felt like Bill Murray in Groundhog Day.

Empty. Measure. Record.
[Oh boy! Here we go again.]

Empty. Measure. Record.
[Are you kidding me?]

Empty. Measure. Record.
[COME ON!!!!]

Empty. Measure. Record.
[I am seriously looking to catch a break here!]

Empty. Measure. Record.
[You have got to be FUCKING kidding me!!!]

The weeks dragged on: 3. . .4. . .5. . .6. . .7.

And little by little my confidence in the process declined. My last vestiges of upbeat state-of-mind and hope for a positive outcome evaporated and my mental state reached what I thought would be my all-time low.

Kind of sad given that I was now considered cancer-free.

At 7 ½ weeks I had a routine visit with Dr. Breast Surgeon that had originally been scheduled to discuss moving on to radiation. And lucky me, I woke up that morning AGAIN running a fever. I was no longer feeling much like a "Lucky Low". I was just feeling LOW.

Hubby escorted me as I was again too sick to drive myself; his wife, who was now fake-strong on the outside, and vulnerable, scared, depressed, disappointed, anxiety-ridden on the inside to see her breast friend. Dr. Breast Surgeon, still the hero, entered the exam room and for the first time I couldn't smile, joke, and be upbeat with him.

He asked, "How are you?"

And I told him straight up, "Not very well."

He opened my gown to take a look and he said, "Oh, this is not good!"

[No shit! You should try to be on this side.]

I looked him right in the eyes and pleadingly asked to have the expanders taken out.

I was done.

I was finally ready to admit defeat and I wanted his help in having it over.

DONE! DONE! DONE!

I was ready to be breastless for the rest of my life. At that moment, I regretted with every cell of my body my decision to have reconstruction. I felt sick. My chest wall hurt all the time from the expanders, my port site was sore, and the tubes inserted into my body had my ribs so sore that reaching for anything was not just uncomfortable but down right painful. And let's not even talk about sleep. That was next to impossible.

At that moment, there was not an ounce of my former badass-self left. Every vestige of that person was gone. And my biggest fear was that it was permanent.

For the first time in my life — a lifetime of being overweight and with a fairly big personality — I felt small. Small and shrunken, like a once ripe apple left out in the sun too long. Not only did I feel shriveled and small, I wanted to just huddle up in a corner, turn into sand, and just be blown away. Dust to dust. I did not want on this ride anymore.

With tears welling up in my eyes, I could see by the concern on Dr. Breast Surgeon's face that he knew I was not in a good place. He may not have been able to relate, but he could certainly empathize, and I loved him even more for that. All I really wanted, at that moment, was for him to let me put my head on his shoulder and just sob. Of course, Jane Wayne would never have allowed that, and even though he was my new breast friend, I knew it wasn't appropriate; but that was just how small and fragile I felt.

Thankfully, he understood where I was, agreed that removing the expanders was probably the right decision to get me on to radiation, and he would call Dr. Plastic Surgeon to arrange what was next. He sent me home with the assurance he would speak with Dr. Plastic Surgeon to schedule ANOTHER surgery and he would call me later that day with the details.

Not feeling any better physically, I felt better that we had a plan.

Later that evening he called me to explain his conversation with Dr. Plastic Surgeon and what they thought the next steps should be. They discussed that if they removed the expanders, I would be right back at square one, as my body would want to refill the newly emptied space again. They decided a better approach was for me to go back to Dr. Plastic Surgeon the next day and he was going to begin to fill the expanders. Although it sounded like a plan, I was actually PISSED! I spent my career in clinical ophthalmology and with some of our procedures, we would insert gas or saline into the eye to fill the space created by the eye surgery we had performed to avoid further problems - like that space filling with fluid the body produced, so it only made sense to do the same with the expanders; fill the space and eventually the body would stop trying to fill that space by creating fluid. At 4 weeks of having the abhorrent drains, I had suggested that to Dr. Plastic Surgeon and his response was, "We just don't do that." And now here we were doing exactly that. I was angry.

Regardless of my anger, I was relieved we now had a plan: fill the bitches as much as I could stand at each appointment, pull the drains and get me back to Dr. Radiation Oncologist as soon as possible.

By this point, cancer (although once the breast tissue and lymph nodes were removed, I was considered free of cancer) had become what felt like a full-time job. All I wanted was to quit this shitty job. Or could I be fired? Someone, please fire me!

With one foot dragging behind the other, I was just a noodle for Hubby to drag to the plastic surgeon. I think he insisted on taking me for fear I might strangle the doctor and finish this journey in prison.

Fortunately, this is where having a high tolerance to pain, and quite literally, little feeling left in my chest, was an advantage. He filled the expanders as much as I could tolerate.

[Bring it on Plastics Boy!]

With a new plan of attack, a little bit of new life had been breathed into Jane Wayne. Shaky, weak, and a bit pissed off at the betrayal of my body, I was now of the mindset to get this done!!!

[Buckle up, Buttercup!]

Empty. Measure. Record.
[Oh my God! Down 10cc's.]

Empty. Measure. Record.
[Are you kidding me? Thank you, baby Jesus!]

Empty. Measure. Record.
[Woohoo!!]

Empty. Measure. Record.
[If it wouldn't hurt so much, I would jump up and down.]

Empty. Measure. Record.
[FUCK YEAH! Call Dr. Plastic Surgeon – let's get these motherfucking drains out of my body! I'm coming off injured reserves!]

One week after starting to fill the expanders, I was back in his office having those despicable tubes pulled out of my sides and had the first half-way decent night's rest in months. I was feeling like a new woman. A battered, used up, tank empty woman. But now I at least felt like we were making progress.

However, the delay in removing the drains had caused a new challenge.

[Go figure!]

To start radiation close to the planned time frame my team had decided upon, Dr. Plastic Surgeon was not going to be able to complete my reconstruction until after the radiation. This was another kick in the ovaries as he shared that radiation was very damaging to the skin and remaining tissues, so the success rate of reconstruction drops significantly, like down to the 50 percentile.

[ARGGGHHH! THAT'S significant!!]

The day after the drains were removed, I was off to see, Dr. Radiation Oncologist. I was ready to start radiation. Radiation that I now considered behind schedule.

[Hop to it. Let's get this going!]

It had been months since I had seen Dr. Radiation Oncologist, and during that time she had moved to a new practice and treatment facility. Fortunately, she was still on my insurance, so I wasn't going to have to look for a different radiation oncologist: I would just need to go to a different location.

We sat down to strategize our radiation plan, certainly different than when we met those many months ago: six weeks of daily radiation, with weekends off for good behavior.

[Alrighty then – let's start tomorrow.]

What everyone needed to know was that I had PLANS; I had someplace I needed to be on May 9. And that was New York for Landry's senior thesis event. Her thesis was creating a fashion collection and participating in a fashion show. The fashion show where she would be presenting her work would be attended by well-known designers, fashion icons, and fashion journalists. This would be the culmination of six years of education: two years in a fashion program at a career and technical high school and four years at The Pratt Institute. And I was going to be there NO MATTER WHAT!

[So, let's get a move-on, Princess!]

If we got started right away, I would be done in time to go.

Dr. Radiation Oncologist explained everything in great detail, answered all my questions, and began a physical exam. Everything was going great until she saw the holes in the side of my ribcage where the drain tubes had been just kinda hanging out for more than seven weeks. Between insertion, removal, re-insertion, and tubes moving around in there for so many weeks, the wounds were open and quite large; large enough that I could have inserted my thumb in the opening, if I was a masochist. Since the initial staph infection, I had become intolerant of Steri-strips (little sticky strips used in place of sutures to hold a wound closed), tape, and Band-Aids. But Dr. Radiation Oncologist is a smart cookie, and she prescribed an old school prescription cream she was sure would heal the wound quickly. She would see me in 10 days.

[Noooooo! I have some place to be. No! No! No! No! No!]
Feeling tears welling up in my eyes, I told her, "Dr. Radiation Oncologist, I HAVE to be in New York by May 9, even if it's just for the day. I need to start this as soon as possible."

[If I can't go, I would rather be dead. NO KIDDING!]

Being there meant EVERYTHING to me.

She assured me that she would do all she could to make that happen and that I just needed to keep reminding her.

Ten days after my initial visit with her, I was back in her office to re-evaluate the wounds and to be temporarily marked for radiation. After a scan (that is not diagnostic but is used for positioning), I was temporarily marked with a Sharpie and clear stickers were placed to cover the marks. They were to remain in place until my next visit, in a week, where I would be tattooed, a mold with my hands over my head would be created (still not the most comfortable position so I was grateful that the mold would hold me in place), and we would go through a dry run of a treatment. I was told that the stickers needed to stay in place and if they didn't, I was to come in and have them redone until the permanent tattoos were placed.

I was also instructed to keep the radiated area as moisturized as possible. That's when I went on an investigative journey to find the best moisturizers, in addition to what they had recommended. After all I had been through, I did not want the rest of my reconstruction to fail so if they told me to put moisturizer on once a day, I was going to double or triple it. I wanted soft supple skin through this. At least THAT I could control.

And all through this I was still having Herceptin infusions, echocardiograms, and bloodwork.

And something very strange, for me, was beginning to occur.

Now, even though I was beginning to see the light at the end of the tunnel, I was starting to lose the thin grasp I had maintained on my mental health. I was in a slump. Mentally, I was falling apart. I was worried about not getting to Landry's fashion show and things were starting to catch up: bills were coming in and it was becoming almost a full-time job to correct some of the mistakes. (I had a blood draw that was mismarked with an Invitro Fertilization code. It took over six months and the billing being sent to collections before I could get it corrected. Someone else's mistake, and no one *willing to correct it and it was now having a negative impact on our credit rating.) Money was flowing out faster than it was coming in. I was starting to have debilitating anxiety attacks, where, if it wasn't for the fact I HAD to go to radiation every day, I was otherwise unable to leave the house.*

And I was too embarrassed to tell anyone. I felt pathetic. Here I was, Jane Wayne, on what I considered the easiest part of this journey and I was falling apart.

But for once, something went my way. My stickers stayed in place, although I was grateful to have them removed as I had become so sensitive to adhesive that those little round circles created by the adhesive remained on my skin as red circles for several weeks.

Twelve days after having my drains removed, I was on the table with my arms over my head listening to the hum of the radiation machine. It took longer to change in and out of my clothes than it did to have a treatment.

[One down; 29 to go.]

After a few days of treatment, I felt even more like I had fallen into a deeper depth of anxiety and depression. All I could do was leave my house for radiation. And even that was hours of convincing myself that I HAD to go. My technician even noticed and suggested I speak with the social worker on staff.

On my next visit, I also saw the social worker. She shared that 90 percent of people going through extended cancer treatment require some medical intervention along the way. I never did look that up to see if it was a factual percentage or not, but I was fully aware that whatever the percentage was, I had reached that point. I was where white-knuckling and clawing through each day, all while being terrified to leave the house, was no longer working for me. Luckily Dr. Radiation

Oncologist was in the office and she wrote me a prescription for Ativan. I was grateful and disappointed at the same time. Grateful that there was something to help but REALLY disappointed that I, Ann Low, aka Jane Wayne, needed help to get through what was now supposed to be the easiest part of the journey. My belief of how strong of a person I was disintegrated with that prescription in my hand.

I sat in my car and cried. And then went straight to the pharmacy.

But there was more to my upset than just everything I had been going through myself. All during this time Terry (my original cancer coach) and I had stayed in touch and were comparing treatment notes. With two wicked senses of humor, we even laughed a lot about where the two of us were at in our treatments. Not all that funny, but it was certainly better than crying about it. Her cancer had spread, and she was flying to Boston to see if she qualified for a clinical trial, her last option for treatment.

She flew to Boston and it looked like she was going to be accepted into the trial. We were thrilled! She would need to be in Boston for treatment two days a week for several months but she could commute and continue her charity work and still have her local medical team here close by and involved.

Just shortly after returning from the visit in Boston she called to tell me she had developed pancreatitis and was in the hospital. Not only did she feel terrible, but it looked like this was going to exclude her from the clinical trial.

I was so sad. We had become close by the commonality of cancer and we spoke, texted, or emailed frequently. I told her I was on my way out to the hospital to see her, and she said, "Please don't. We'll get together as soon as I'm out of the hospital, but please don't come here and expose yourself to all the germs and things here." I reluctantly agreed, but I was unhappy about it.

But she didn't come home from the hospital. Not long after our call, one of her close friends called to tell me they were moving her to hospice. I said that I was on my way, but Terry was adamant that she didn't want any visitors other than family members and those that were already there with her. I TOTALLY understood, but I was devastated.

I suddenly realized that I was going to lose my mentor and the world was going to lose Terry.

And two days later she was gone. My mentor. My coach. My friend.

[FUCK CANCER!! Fuck every bit of this! FUCK. FUCK. FUCK.]

Just days later the father of one of my son's friends succumbed to his cancer.

My heart felt squishy and my eyes leaked. I felt sad for everyone involved; including myself. It was all fresh and in my face, and I hated every moment of the injustice of the cancer deaths I was now so acutely aware of.

I hated cancer so much!

The rest of radiation treatment was pretty straight forward. I had a routine I followed to try and keep my skin as moisturized as possible. I went back to an old cracked skin remedy from years ago (lanolin) and Aquaphor. Lanolin is a wax secreted by wool-bearing animals and is referred to as wool fat. It has natural waterproofing that helps sheep in shedding water from their wool and is used widely in high-value cosmetics and skin treatment products. I used the lanolin at night and anytime I didn't have to leave the house, and I used the

Aquaphor any time I had to leave the house, mainly because I didn't want to walk around smelling like a wooly sheep.

I knew this regimen was working when one morning I woke up to an array of blisters and scabs on the upper left quadrant of my back. I'm not sure if I missed it, if someone forgot to tell me, or it didn't seem important at the time, but I learned on that day that I had an exit pathway for the radiation and my upper shoulder now looked like what I was worried my chest would look like. Good news: my chest was a nice healthy WHITE, soft, and not "sunburned." Bad news: my back was not. I went home and began the same treatment on my back and although my back stayed sunburned throughout the rest of radiation, my chest stayed moist, healthy, and free of any side effects.

Radiation typically has two side effects: skin changes and fatigue. I felt like I had the skin changes under control and I wasn't feeling any fatigue.

As a matter of fact, I was beginning to feel stronger every day. I was back to walking, although I knew I wasn't ready to go back to the gym just yet. Between the expanders, and my port rubbing on my sternum, the last thing I wanted to do was anything that required use of chest muscles.

I began to feel even more smug as radiation neared the end, my skin was still fine, AND we had figured out a schedule that would allow me to go to Landry's fashion show in New York. Of course, there were new precautions: a sleeve to prevent lymphedema for when I flew, Clorox wipes to wipe every surface I would touch on the plane, and skin sanitizer that I found myself practically washing my hands in every five minutes.

[Yes, I had become a bit of a germaphobe.]

With 91-year-old FIL and Hubby, we traveled to Brooklyn for Landry's event. For the first time since Aug. 4, 2014, I don't think I thought about my cancer but a few times while we were there. I could enjoy the trip, my daughter's beautiful creations, celebrate her recognition and scholarship from Rolls Royce, and attend a Roll Royce event where they rolled out their new model of car and honored my daughter for her craftsmanship. Dressed in one of her beautiful designs, surrounded by famous and influential people, with Hubby and FIL by my side, I felt like a million bucks.

In the blink of an eye, I was back on a plane, back in the sleeve, wiping away germs, and sanitizing every few minutes.

I returned for five more days of radiation, received my graduation certificate, and continued with appointments with Mom, FIL, Herceptin, bloodwork, and an occasional echocardiogram. Now it was just a matter of regaining my strength, bitching about the expanders, and letting my radiated skin heal the six months required before we would exchange the expanders for the implants and I had been released to finally schedule a colonoscopy which I eventually had and it showed polyps that I had biopsied and removed but, THANKFULLY, did NOT show any cancer.

I could see the end in sight.

[FINALLY.]

Then some, what seemed like little, unusual things began to happen. First, I noticed that, every time I stood up, I felt so light headed I thought I would pass out. I decided to start checking my blood pressure and it would be 100/60 or lower. However, my resting heart rate, which is normally around 70, was 125 bpm.

[Hmmmm? That's weird!]

Then I started running a low-grade fever.

[Really? You have got to be kidding me!]

This went on for a couple days. Then I noticed it was getting harder to walk as I was experiencing shortness of breath.

[Huh. I guess all that Cloroxing and sanitizing did a WHOLE lot of good! Guess I'm going to get sick. Dammit!]

Then one afternoon I sat down to read some work paperwork. I closed my eyes...just for a moment...and woke up two hours later.

[Whaaat? Now I'm going to have the radiation fatigue AND be sick?]

I just kept an eye on it for a few days figuring it was just a bug that needed to run its course, but I was feeling pretty crappy.

Then one morning, on my walk, something happened. I got halfway through my walk when I became so short of breath I had to stop and bend over to try and get oxygen into my lungs, and my heart was pounding so hard you could see it through my shirt. I knew it was time to call Dr. Medical Oncologist.

Within an hour I was in and out of the oncologist's office and on my way to a CAT scan and chest X-ray. Soon after came a call from Dr. Medical Oncologist letting me know that thankfully my cancer had not spread and but that the radiologist had determined I had pneumonia.
[Well that certainly explains things!]

With the busiest time of the year for Little League now beginning, I was anxious to get to feeling better, so I could participate. I followed the doctor's orders and took my antibiotics and did what my body would let me do, which was very little. I had an annoying cough, shortness of breath, I just about passed out every time I stood up, my resting heart rate was still consistently over 125 bpm, and I was still running a low-grade fever.

A week later, after a follow-up chest X-Ray, I was back in Dr. Medical Oncologist's office. I felt no better, but per the radiologist, my X-Ray was clear. However, with still being symptomatic, Dr. Medical Oncologist decided to change the antibiotics, send me for an echocardiogram, and have me see a cardiologist

I saw Dr. Medical Oncologist on Monday, had a routine follow-up with Dr. Breast Surgeon on Tuesday, had a routine visit with Dr. Radiation Oncologist on Wednesday, and was scheduled with my new addition, Dr. Cardiologist, on Thursday and my mom had an appointment with her cardiologist along in there as well.

Things took a bit of a turn when that Friday I had a routine follow-up with Dr. Radiation Oncologist. When she saw me, she said, "You don't look like you feel very well." I replied, "I don't. This is week two of being treated for pneumonia." She got a quizzical look on her face and asked me what my symptoms were. After hearing what was going on, she told me that she actually did not think I had pneumonia and that she wanted to examine the X-rays and CAT scan, then she would call me later.

Later that evening, she called and told me that she thought I had something called Radiation Pneumonitis.
[Oh boy – something new and exciting with silent letters to add to this journey.]

Radiation pneumonitis is a side effect of radiation therapy that involves the lungs. While radiation is used to damage cancer cells and to stop them from growing and dividing, it is inevitable that normal cells can also be affected. The lungs can become inflamed and this is termed radiation pneumonitis.

She suggested that I keep my appointment the next day with Dr. Cardiologist to rule out any heart problems, given that Herceptin can cause congestive heart failure, but she felt pretty certain my issue was my lungs, not my heart.

The next day I saw Dr. Cardiologist, who assured me that upon first examination it seemed like my ticker was ticking appropriately. But like all good doctors, he wanted to be sure so we better repeat the EKG and echocardiogram.

[Kaching!]

(Rant ahead! I call this insistence on doing every test possible, defensive medicine. We have become such a litigious society that a doctor must send you for every freaking test just to cover their asses (and assets). More tests; higher costs for treatment and insurance. The vicious cycle of our broken health care system.)

All the while, I'm still feeling crappy and my afternoon naps have become a daily necessity. I'm now sleeping two to four hours in the afternoon and eight to 10 hours at night, and yet, still feeling so exhausted I can barely function.

Two weeks after Dr. Radiation Oncologist shared her opinion with me, and Dr. Cardiologist confirmed my ticker was in excellent health, Dr. Medical Oncologist decided it was time for me to visit ANOTHER new doctor, Dr. Pulmonologist.
At this point, Little League tournaments had gotten under way, and I made it to opening night, which is always an exciting time: little guys with oversized gloves and bats that seem longer than they are tall, and rock star older players wanting to make it to Williamsport to play on ESPN. Opening

night. Sunflower seeds and the crack of that bat on the ball. A night I love!

But that was far as I got. Feeling light-headed, short of breath, having difficulty swallowing, still running a low-grade fever every day, and needing multiple hours of naps, I was in no condition to be out at the baseball fields every night.

I was in no condition to be anywhere but on my couch.

I hated it.

Dr. Pulmonologist saw me, and I gave him my history, including the opinion of Dr. Radiation Oncologist. After looking at my X-ray and CAT scan, he decided that it still could be pneumonia and that one more regimen of antibiotics was warranted. Then we would do another CAT scan and if there were no definitive changes, he would schedule me for a lung biopsy.

[REALLY??!!!]

And all during this time I'm still having Herceptin, bloodwork, and taking Mom, FIL and MIL to doctor appointments. Oh, and taking naps. Lots of naps.

After my follow-up CAT scan, I was back in Dr. Pulmonologist's office, where he agreed that I had radiation pneumonitis. The diffuse changes I had in my lungs were now more defined and certainly supported the case for my lungs being inflamed rather than infected.

[Well at least that only took 7 weeks to figure out!]

With a definitive diagnosis, there also became a definitive treatment: oral steroids. I wasn't worried about the steroids as we were only going to be using them for six weeks. What harm could that cause? And if it meant I would finally start to feel better, I was all for it. I was sick and tired of being sick and tired. I just wanted to start feeling better at a time when most people were well into recovery.

I began my steroids and within days began to feel better.

Self-Care

Although cancer is a team sport, YOU must be the one to step up to the plate to swing at the pitches that are thrown your way.

Occasionally, you may unexpectedly get beaned with a curveball.

I remember the first time my son was hit by a pitch and was hurting, the first base coach met him and said, "Rub some dirt on it."

Sometimes it's difficult to know just where to rub that dirt as cancer is such a rollercoaster ride. Bad news. Good news. No news.

Regardless of how great your cancer care team is, with its doctors and your support squad, being diagnosed with cancer and undergoing treatment can impact your mental well-being.

[Really? Say it isn't so!]

A cancer diagnosis is a life-altering event. Not only are you trying to cope with the diagnosis, you are also still in the game of life. The everyday stresses of life don't just disappear because you have cancer. It feels like the world should stop, but the sun will still come up in the East and set in the West. Your lender will still want you to pay your mortgage. Your ex might still be a jerk. Your kids will still spill Kool-Aid in the kitchen. Your dog still needs to be walked. The garbage barrel still needs to go out to the street. Your cat may still hack up a hairball on the carpet. Other family members may get sick.

Life goes on.

A certain amount of distress is normal when you have cancer. With that distress, can be some amazing mood swings. Anesthesia, medications, chemotherapy, radiation, surgery, and many other things can also contribute to these swings in your emotions.

Andrew H. Miller, M.D., the Director of Psychiatric Oncology at the Winship Cancer Institute at Emory University School of Medicine, says that cancer and most cancer treatments can activate the immune system to release inflammatory cytokines. That's medical speak for these little chemical messengers, released into your cells, that signal to increase or decrease inflammation. He states, "Research has shown that inflammatory cytokines can enter the brain and affect many of the brain circuits and chemicals that are involved in depression, anxiety, fatigue and impairment in memory and concentration."

This is where self-care becomes so important. Finding things to make the experience as pleasant as possible for yourself will help. That sometimes isn't easy, as you go through the roller coaster of treatment and emotions, but there are many things that can help.

About the time I was due to start radiation, my ability to cope with the emotional rollercoaster of cancer began to slip through my neuropathy-plagued fingers. A little one day. More the next. Coming from multi-generations of familial crazies, I just assumed the chemo had triggered the family genes into action.

What I later found out from a social worker was that many, many cancer patients struggle with depression and anxiety during treatment.

If you find that you are having these issues, tell your doctor about your feelings. If needed, they will refer you to someone who can help you through talk therapy, medication or both.

One suggestion I received was that I consider joining a Support Group. I was not very open to the idea in the beginning. That's actually not true. I was ADAMANT it was not for me, and never would be.

[Whaaat?? I'm Jane Wayne (the female version of John Wayne – circle the wagons, save the women and children, chase off the enemy and then come back to whup up some tasty grub.) I don't need no stinkin' help. I became sober without a Support Group . . . I'm pretty damn sure I can DO cancer without one!]

Boy, was I ever wrong!

I shared the recommendation that I consider joining a support group with Hubby; he thought it was a fabulous idea. Me – not so much! With great support and encouragement from him, I reluctantly agreed to go to ONE meeting, and if I didn't like it I didn't HAVE to go back.

The day of the meeting arrived, and I grudgingly drove to the meeting site. I sat in my car in the parking lot. I walked part way to the door and went back to my car. Finally, I realized I was a big girl and all growed up and if I didn't like it I could just pick up my things and leave. I didn't have to stay.

I went expecting it to be all doom and gloom. It was nothing like that. It was so supportive to be with a group of people that have either traveled the road before you, are going through it as well, or are also new to the cancer journey. Finally, here was a place to talk about my experiences and concerns with others; feelings I felt too strange to share with my, at home, non-cancer teammates.

Sitting in that room, with those amazing women – all with their own individual stories, yet all of us connected by a common thread – that bitch known as breast cancer – I felt the stress melt a little for the very first time. It was cathartic. It felt healing. For the first time in a long time, it helped me feel more in control as I would listen to others and say in my head, "You mean I'm not the only one?" It was if a giant weight had been lifted off my shoulders and I had a safe place to "be" with my cancer.

Not only did I learn a lot, and I developed some amazing friendships, I was, and still am, most stunned as others came up to me to tell me what an inspiration I was for them! Me? An inspiration? I never thought that; but how refreshing to know you can have had a positive impact on someone just with your presence there. Now, there is **nothing** that keeps me from these meetings.

Support Groups: Groups are offered across the country in a variety of ways. You will want to find the group that works best for you. Here are some of the different options of support groups:
- Peer-led groups are facilitated by group members; usually someone who has had your type of cancer.
- Professional-led groups are led by a trained counselor, psychologist or social worker.
- Informational support groups are usually led by a professional facilitator who invites expert speakers such as doctors, nurse navigators, nutritionists or others who provide expert advice.

Groups can also be for specific audiences, such as:
- All individuals with cancer.
- People with a specific type of cancer.
- Certain age groups, like teens or children.
- Caregivers. (This journey is as hard, in some cases harder, on the ones who love and care for us. They need support too!)

In the age of technology, Internet support groups have gained popularity. These are great options for people who live too far away to get to a meeting, have challenges with transportation, are not comfortable sharing in person or are too ill to travel to a meeting. These support groups can also connect people with rare types of cancer to each other.

Internet groups communicate in a variety of ways:
- Email lists: send messages written by group members that get sent out to the entire group.
- Discussion groups, message boards or bulletin boards allow people to post a message that others can reply to.
- Chat rooms: these allow members to communicate with each other by typing messages back and forth in real time.

How to find a support group:
- Check with your doctor or treatment facility. Many offer their patients support groups at the treatment center.
- Internet. Search using "Support Group" with your type of cancer.
- Ask other patients.
- CancerCare.org – Search Support Group.
- National Cancer Institute — Search Support Group.

• • •

Massage: Cancer treatment is an arduous process. Massage therapy can help with pain or stress relief during this time. You will want to make sure you okay any massage therapy with your doctor prior to having one. Here are some suggestions to consider if your doctor tells you that a massage is fine for you during treatment:

- Whenever possible locate a Massage Therapist that has been trained in cancer massage. To locate a practitioner near you; go to The Society for Oncology Massage website at www.s4om.org.
- If you cannot find an Oncology Massage Therapist, be sure to ask your doctor if they have a recommendation.
- Be sure to ask your team if you have any restrictions for a massage such as not being able to lie on your stomach or avoiding radiation treatment areas.
- Avoid deep tissue massage, hot stones, exfoliation treatments and herbal wraps.

• • •

Exercise: I know. I know. I keep mentioning it. But it made such a difference for me that I think it should be one of the top things on your list of self-care items. This is NOT the time to start training for a marathon or joining the new CrossFit gym. But it is the time to move your body. LISTEN to your body and find what works for you. Know that it may fluctuate through treatment. Most days I could hike or walk 3 to 5 miles, but there were days that I only made it to the mailbox and back. REALLY listen to your body. As my oncologist said, "It will let you know what you can do."

• • •

Meet with a Nutritionist: Nutrition can be an important part of cancer treatment and is especially important after treatment is completed and you move into survivorship. Meeting with a nutritionist can support you in knowing the right foods, liquids and even possibly the best supplements to assist you with your fight against cancer and any negative side effects.

- Ask at your treatment center. More centers are adding whole body approaches in their treatment centers, with many of them having a nutritionist on staff.
- Search the Internet: Use "Cancer Nutritionist" and the city you reside in and it will give you options. If there are none in your area, you may find an online nutritionist to assist you.
- Check with your insurance company. Many companies offer nutritional services as part of their health and wellness programs.
- American Dietetic Association: Click on the button "Find a Nutritionist."

• • •

Dry Brushing: Dry brushing stimulates the body's circulation and lymphatic systems. The lymphatic system is a pretty lazy structure in our body and yet is responsible for waste removal via your lymph nodes. Dry brushing can not only brush off dead skin cells, but also stimulate the lymphatic system and body to shed excess cellular waste products. (Besides the fact that it feels pretty darn good, too!) This is where dry brushing can be invaluable, as lymphatic congestion is a major factor leading to inflammation.

- Get a long handled natural bristled brush. These can be found at health food stores, vitamin shops or online.

(Always okay with your physician first; especially if you have lymphedema.)

- The best time to do it is first thing in the morning before you shower but it can be done anytime.
- Start at your ankles and brush upward using light to firm strokes. Brush several times in each area, overlapping as you go.
- When brushing, brush toward your heart, which is best for circulation and your lymphatic system. Your skin might be pink but should not hurt. If it does, you are brushing too hard.
- Brushing can last as little as two minutes, or up to twenty, so it is easy to add to your daily regimen.
- Drink a glass of room temperature water (lemon slice optional) to get your digestive system going after dry brushing.

• • •

Find an activity: Many of the cancer treatments centers have expanded to include additional resources other than just medical treatment. Studies indicate that addressing your psychological and spiritual health can help in the recovery process and in future prevention. Some of these complementary programs and therapies might include:

- Healing art
- Journaling classes
- Hatha yoga
- Yoga nidra
- Qi gong
- Tia chi
- Reiki
- Meditation
- Relaxation techniques

- Book clubs

• • •

Medical Therapy: Sometime none of these self-care suggestions are enough to treat the emotions that might impact you during this time. If that becomes the case, you should seek counseling or therapy to assist you in dealing with any feelings you may be experiencing such as anxiety, depression, anger, guilt and confusion. Many doctors encourage their patients to seek out a therapist to cope with their diagnosis.

- **Oncology Social Workers:** With special training to help people cope with the diagnosis, oncology social workers can help individuals better understand the health care system and provide them with options through their treatment. Many treatment centers now have Oncology Social Workers on staff.
- **Psychologist:** Psychologists receive graduate training in psychology and are trained to talk patients through their challenges.
- **Psychiatrist:** Like psychologists, psychiatrists are also trained to talk with patients about their challenges, but they are also medical doctors, so they can prescribe medication. They might find medications necessary after assessing a patient for other contributing factors such as vitamin deficiencies or thyroid problems.
- **Family Counseling:** Sometimes it is of great value to have family counseling. Cancer really does affect every member of the family and for some, having an outside source guide them through the unique challenges of a family member with cancer can be quite beneficial.

Finding a good connection with a counselor is as important as knowing about their training. You may have to talk with several potential counselors before finding one that feels best for you and/or your family.

Tips for finding a counselor:
- Ask about the services offered at your cancer treatment center or hospital.
- Ask your doctors for referrals.
- Ask members of your cancer support group.
- Internet search.

Be sure to check with your insurance company for coverage. There are plenty of options for self-care during cancer therapy. Self-care can provide some great balance and perspective on whether to duck if you think a ball is coming right at you or to swing hard, follow-through and try to take one to the fence in this game of cancer.

• • •

Tips:

- Ask yourself about your self-care skills. "Do I take care of myself last? "If so, NOW is the time to change that. (You can always do that once you get to survivorship, if you choose.) You need to be somewhat selfish in taking care of yourself and communicating it effectively to your support team.
- Set boundaries: No calls before 10:00 AM. No visitors the week after chemo. No drop-in visitors. Whatever works best for you. Set boundaries and stick to them.
- Designate someone to be your communicator. Usually your primary care giver will be that person. I utilized Hubby to call all the family and our closest friends after surgeries or any other important events.

- Try to eliminate stress. Find ways to reduce stress during this time, or ways to respond differently.
- Sleep. ZZZZZZZZZZZZZZZZZZZZZZ. Sleep is one of the greatest natural healers. Now is the time to adjust your schedule to get as much sleep as possible.
- Stop "SHOULDING" all over yourself. Most of the stuff we tell ourselves we SHOULD be doing will be there tomorrow, next week or even next month. If it MUST get done and you are unable, enlist your support squad.

• • •

My Story:

I could slowly begin walking again, my fever began to fade, I was less tired, and my blood pressure and heart rate began to return to normal. My confidence in myself and my medical team began to improve as I felt I was back on the road to recovery.

Then three weeks into the high dose steroid regiment for the radiation pneumonitis things began to feel off. In just the three short weeks, I had gained 20 pounds from the steroids and my anxiety was back with a vengeance. Actually, it was so bad I was canceling appointments and engagements. I was trapped in my head and in my house. I was falling head first down the rabbit hole of anxiety and depression. If it wasn't a Herceptin infusion or doctor appointment, I could barely drag myself anywhere. I told Hubby I was going places and doing things when in reality I was barely going outside.

Ande then one day I woke up so sad, depressed and despondent that I knew there was absolutely no value to me staying on the planet. As much as I am embarrassed and ashamed to admit it, I was suicidal. I knew the best thing for everyone involved would be for me to end my life. No more mounting medical debt. No more pain or medication. I knew with every cell of my body that with my life insurance, I was more valuable dead than alive. House paid off. College debt gone. And no more pain in the ass daughter, sister, mother, friend or wife to have to worry about. I didn't feel like I could tell anyone, as I felt I had already been such a horrible burden to my family emotionally, physically and economically. How do you tell the people you love you are going to kill yourself? Especially when the journey is almost over.

[Hey – just sorta thinking about ending my life! No biggie – right?!]

With my family gone, I searched for the 9mm Hubby had somewhere. Able to find it in my frantic search, but unable to find any ammunition and I just stood in the kitchen sobbing

But from the depth of that despair, I remembered what Terry had been suggesting I do for months. With what little rational thought I had left, I called her psychiatrist and told his receptionist I was suicidal. They had no appointment openings, but they suggested I get to the emergency room as soon as possible. I doubled up on my Ativan, which was like putting a Band-Aid on a mortal wound and I made myself go outside. At least outside, I knew I was safe from myself. Again, I found myself on my patio swing.

Hours later Hubby returned from work and right away he could tell I was not doing very well. I told him that I was on the shakiest ground I had ever been on and that he might need to take me to the hospital. My recollection was that I told him it was because I was afraid I was going to kill myself. He says I never said that part; that all I said was that I might need him to take me to the hospital. Regardless, I made it through the night without going to the hospital or without taking my life.

[Obviously!]

And the Luck of the Lows showed up. The psychiatrist's office called me early that next morning. They had a cancellation, and did I still want to come in?

In less than an hour I was sitting in front of Dr. Make Me Uncrazy. I told him all that was going on, and when we got to what medications I was on he shared with me that it was possible for high dose steroids to cause some people to have psychiatric symptoms which was known as Steroid Psychosis.

[Great! A psychotic episode!]

However weird it might sound; it was a relief to know it was the Prednisone. At least there was a reason. And since I was slowly being tapered off it for the Radiation Pneumonitis, that meant there was hope! I just needed to hang on while the Prednisone was tapered, and the anti-depressants and anti-anxiety medications began to work.

And I did hang on. White knuckled. Hanging by a thread; by only my nails. Lost in a world that was so scary that I now needed to have Hubby take me to the doctors as I didn't trust myself behind the wheel as sometimes oncoming traffic looked inviting.

As the Prednisone was tapered and the make me not crazy medications began to do their thing, I began to feel a little better each day. A little stronger. Certainly, far from the person I was before August of 2014, but I was no longer yearning for life to all be over. Cancer treatment, yes; life – no.

And then September 10th arrived, and I had my last Herceptin infusion. A year of chemotherapy and antibody therapy was over. Funny — at times it seemed like it had just started and at other times I felt like I had been doing this for years.

For me it was pretty anti-climactic. I still had expanders in, so I had at least one more surgery. I may be cancer-free, I may have made it through chemotherapy and radiation, but I still had more treatment ahead and this left me feeling like things just weren't done yet.

And I was still on shaky ground. So, I began to research something that I never thought I would do; I began to consider support groups.

I never saw myself as a support group kind of person, but I was still feeling incredibly unstable. I hurt. I needed a nap every day. I could be in the middle of a conversation and completely forget what I was saying. I felt like a completely different person. And in October of 2015 I didn't have the faintest clue who that person was. I knew I wasn't my cancer; I had cancer, but it didn't have me. But I was still unsure of myself and not sure who I could share those feelings with. With trembling hands, I began a search for a local Breast Cancer Support group.

*And wouldn't you know it there was one **THAT** Saturday; nice and close. Ugh. I told Hubby I was thinking about going, but I wasn't very excited about it. He thought it was a brilliant idea.*

On Saturday, I forced myself into my car, imagining nothing but depressing and morose stories sprinkled in with plenty of crying and complaining. I was already depressed and I don't tolerate complaining very well; I just couldn't imagine that there would be anything positive there for me.

I pulled into a parking spot and just sat there in my running car. Then I backed my car out of the spot and started to leave.

[Shit!]

Then I pulled back into the parking spot. I even left my car to go in the building, but made it only half-way there before I turned back to my car. With my car unlocked and my door half open, I finally said to myself, "Ann, you are 53 years old and you are a big girl. Go in to the meeting. If you hate it, get up and leave."

With trembling hands and a racing heart, I forced myself into the building and went to the meeting room where the support group would meet. There were already several women gathered, waiting to enter the locked room. They were smiling and hugging and seemed happy. I stood off to the side and watched. Some were bald, some had on hats or scarves, but most had full heads of hair and looked quite radiant and as if they were thriving. Soon a woman came up by my side and welcomed me. She could tell that I was nervous, and I could feel myself on the verge of tears while my belly was rebelling with nausea. She shared that she had been coming for years and that she hoped I found as much value out of the group as most people did.

The doors opened and we all moved in and sat down.

At this particular support group, which was a peer led group, we went around the room, introduced ourselves, gave a brief description of our date of diagnosis and what treatments we had received thus far. I was surprised to hear there were people that were long time survivors and had been coming for years and others that were newly diagnosed. Once we went around the room the facilitator then asked if anyone had something they wanted to talk about. These women, of all different ages and stages, shared things they were going through.

THINGS I WAS GOING THROUGH!

[HOLY CRAP!!! You too??? It's not just me?]

Tears started to gently roll down my face. Not tears of sadness. Not tears of depression. Tears of relief. I had found a place where we all spoke the same language.

[OH MY GOD WHY DID I WAIT SO LONG??!!]

I left that meeting knowing two things for certain: 1) I felt better than I had in MONTHS; 2) If I wasn't traveling, I was going to be at every Support Group Meeting, from that point forward. Non-negotiable. (I now tell every cancer patient that reaches out to me, to get to one as soon as possible.)

Once the Herceptin infusions were complete, I was scheduled for what was called a "Survivor's" visit with my oncologist. More cancer treatment centers and private practices are scheduling these types of appointments often called Survivorship Care Plans. These plans include guidelines for monitoring and maintaining your health. They include details of your treatment, give you information to help you discuss post treatment needs with your primary care physician (who at this point becomes your primary care giver again), cover side effects of any ongoing medications you might need to take, and develop a plan of post treatment follow-up care. This, to me, is a great service and I hope all cancer practices eventually do it. It gave me information to identify symptoms of recurrence and it spelled out the appointments I would require in the future, so I could make an informed decision about my insurance coverage, given that my insurance coverage has changed each year since 2009.

But being handed my Survivorship Care Plan did not leave me with any of the feelings I thought I would have. From the beginning of this crazy ride, I was sure that when they told me not to come back for three months, I would have been doing a happy dance. When the, Nurse Practitioner, covered the plan and said, "I'll see you in three months," I said, "Thank you."

HOWEVER, the little voice inside my head was far less receptive.

[Oh no, no, NO! You have been seeing me every week for a year. You are going to keep seeing me! I am not going away for 3 months. What if we missed something? Nope. Nope. Nope. Nope. Nope.]

Funny thing – almost every survivor I've spoken to about it felt the same way.

It was like when my first husband told me he wasn't in love with me, and never had been and that marrying me had been a big mistake. There was this void that I had NO idea how to fill. I, again, felt this way when Dr. Medical Oncologist told me to go away for three months. It just felt so wrong! SO Scary. Good lord, what had become of my bad-ass self?

[Could I just come sit in the waiting room? Please give me another chance. Maybe I could just sit in the parking lot. I promise to be a better patient. How about I come back in two weeks? Are you hiring? I could sweep the floors or something. PLEASE DON'T MAKE ME GO!!!!]

Dr. Medical Oncologist may have needed a break to "see other people". But I didn't. I felt discombobulated.

But soon I ended up filling my time by receiving Oncology Rehabilitation and Physical Therapy and so the pain of the separation was replaced with the pain of physical therapy. I had gotten to a point that I could not straighten the surgical side arm or lift it above my head because of "lymphatic cording." Cording can sometimes occur after lymph nodes have been removed. It feels like a ropelike structure under the skin of your inner arm. These tend to be painful and tight and make it difficult for you to lift your arm any higher than your *shoulder or allow you to extend your elbow fully. Other than that, it's no big deal. (wink, wink!)*

[Cancer – the gift that just keeps on giving!]

(If you find you need physical therapy due to movement restrictions post treatment, try to find someone trained in Oncology Physical Therapy. Physical Therapists trained in Oncology Rehabilitation have a much more comprehensive understanding of some of the deeper physiological impacts of cancer on the body's system and how their specialized training can lessen some of this impact.)

I was also scheduled to return to Dr. Plastic Surgeon to discuss and perhaps schedule the completion of my reconstruction. There was beginning to be a glimmer of a light at the end of the tunnel and it no longer looked like an oncoming train.

With my radiated skin looking good and feeling soft, the date for my last reconstruction procedure was now on the books. I had decided long before that I was going to forgo having nipples done. Dr. Plastic Surgeon had explained in the beginning that it was the one surgery that could have complications and infections. Given my history of staph infections, all I could picture was one day standing in the shower and them coming off and washing down the drain. And it's not like I needed them anymore. I decided I would be a part of Free the Nipples Campaign; maybe not quite like those freeing them to breast feed, but mine were certainly free.

On October 26th, in an outpatient procedure, I had the expanders replaced with cute little perky implants. I was also going to be deported. Perky implants and rid of the port. I was more than ready!

For once, things went smoothly – with no complications. (It helped that I pretreated my skin and took antibiotics prior to and after the surgery. Sometimes you have to continue to advocate for yourself and your health!)

The relief of having the expanders out was such a respite that, even though I had been cut open, AGAIN, I wanted to jump for joy. I still had areas on my ribs and sternum that were sore and my pectoral muscles on my radiated side were scarred, these things seem minor compared to the ongoing, constant pain of the expanders and the port that I felt was trying to figure out how to claw its way out of my body.

Recovery went well and, in what seemed like a blink of an eye, it was the end of December and I was released from Dr. Plastic Surgeon as well.

Walk off home run!!!

But there was no dog pile. No pennant. No champagne drinking from the trophy. It was just done. Over.

I actually didn't know what to do with myself. I was done with Physical Therapy, all my surgeries, chemo and radiation were over, and I felt . . . well . . . kind of lost. Now all my doctors had broken up with me. There would be some visitation every three months for a year and those appointments would get further apart the longer I was free of disease, but I felt like . . . now what?

I sat in my car and just kind of shook my head. What does it look like after you win the World Series and all the parties are over?

Survivorship (Post Mortem)

I've always found it strange that when the coaches take their team off to the side to dissect the game, win or lose, it's called a post-mortem. It just sounds so terminal. Post-Mortem literally means an examination of a dead body to determine the cause of death. So even if you win it's called a post-mortem?? Seems strange to me. Shouldn't it be called something else if you win?

But here I am in the post-mortem (survivorship) of my 16 inning (months) game of cancer.

My team won and I'm refusing any rematch.

So, now what?

That's what you are currently holding in your hands.

I honestly didn't plan to write a book.

I didn't plan to become an advocate for other cancer patients.

I didn't plan on becoming such an outspoken advocate about cancer prevention and how we must all take personal responsibility and charge of our health.

I didn't plan on co-founding a venture fund that invests in early-stage cancer innovations (www.cancerfund.com). We are erroneously led to believe we must invest more in cancer research to end cancer. Actually, cancer research is VERY well funded. What's missing is funding for viable preventions, diagnostics and therapeutics that come from that well-funded research and become products that can benefit patients. THAT'S what needs more funding and why we started Cancer Fund.

And yet, here I am doing all these things.

The last thing that Terry said to me on that first day we met to discuss what lay ahead, was that cancer would change me and that if she and I were to sit down a year from that conversation she bet that I would tell her that was true. And that she was pretty sure I would tell her that it was a change for the better. At that time, I could not even fathom what that could possibly mean.

Now, to say that cancer has changed my life would be an understatement.

I've realized that this journey was not a battle; I don't do confrontations or battle well. This was just life, which is often brutally random and unfair and that's simply how it goes sometimes.

"Everything happens for a reason." That's the kind of bullshit that destroys lives and it's untrue. And worst of all that keeps us from doing the one thing we must do when our lives are turned upside down: grieve. The reality: some things in life cannot be fixed — they can only be carried.

While loss has made me acutely aware and empathetic to the pains of others, it's also makes me more inclined to sometimes hide out. I have a more cynical view of human nature and a greater impatience with people unfamiliar with what loss does to people.

I'm becoming more used to the fact that fear of recurrence is part of the contract I never agreed to sign, to the club I never asked to join, that has a lifetime membership.

My one hope, with this book, is that it will aid you as you begin this journey — to make it just a little bit easier for you. If something I shared in this book makes it just a little bit easier for just one person, it will have been worth putting in the time it has taken to write this.

"Terry, we didn't get to have that coffee a year down the road, but you were right. Cancer changed me forever and I feel it has been changed for the better."

And I'm fairly certain that it will change you too. But it's up to you to decide what that change will mean in your life and who you will become as a result.

For me, this is not the end, or even the beginning of the end. For me this is just the end of the beginning.

In completing this book, it's my hope that it has been of value to you and that you feel more empowered as you head off to face whatever is in YOUR base path. I hope you utilize the information to be your own advocate or to make sure you find someone who will advocate with or for you.

But mostly I hope you feel better equipped to go out there to kick cancer's ass and swing for the fences! ♥♥♥

Cancer Resources

General Information and Support

AliveAndKickn
www.aliveandkickn.org

American Cancer Society
https://www.cancer.org

American Cancer Society Cancer Survivors Network
http://csn.cancer.org

American Society of Clinical Oncology
www.cancer.net

Annie Appleseed Project
https://www.annieappleseedproject.org

Association of American Cancer Institutes
https://www.aaci-cancer.org/

Association of Cancer Online Resources
www.acor.org

Bag It Cancer
https://bagitcancer.org/

Be The Match
https://bethematch.org

Biomarker Collaborative

https://biomarkercollaborative.org

Bone Marrow & Cancer Foundation
https://bonemarrow.org

Cactus Cancer Society
https://cactuscancer.org

Cancer Care
https://www.cancercare.org

Cancer Commons
https://cancercommons.org

Cancer Core Recovery
https://cancercorerecovery.org

Cancer Dudes
https://cancerdudes.org

Cancer Hope Network
www.cancerhopenetwork.org

Cancer Support Community
www.cancersupportcommunity.org

Caring Connections
www.caringinfo.org

Chemocare
https://chemocare.com/

COA Patient Advocacy Network (CPAN)

https://coaadvocacy.org

Cook For Your Life
https://www.cookforyourlife.org

Cooking for Chemo
https://www.cookingforchemo.org

Exon 20 Group
https://exon20group.org

Expect Miracles Foundation
https://www.expectmiraclesfoundation.org

Florida Cancer Specialists Foundation
https://fcsf.org

Fuck Cancer
https://www.letsfcancer.com

GRYT
https://gryhealth.com

International Cancer Advocacy Network (ICAN)
https://askican.org

Life with Cancer
https://www.lifewithcancer.org

KRAS Kickers
https://www.kraskickers.org

Maureen's Hope Foundation

https://www.maureenshope.org

National Cancer Institute
www.cancer.gov

National Coalition for Cancer Survivorship
www.canceradvocacy.org

OncoLink
https://www.oncolink.org

Patient Empowerment Network
http://www.powerfulpatients.org

Prevent Cancer Foundation
https://www.preventcancer.org

Resilientship
https://www.resilientship.com

Rio Grande Cancer Foundation
https://rgcf.org

Scott Hamilton Cares Foundation
https://www.scottcares.org

The Angiogenesis Foundation
https://angio.org/

The Half Fund
https://thehalffund.org

24 Foundation

https://www.24foundation.org

V Foundation
https://www.v.org

VHL Alliance
https://www.vhl.org

Vital Options
https://www.vitaloptions.org

Caregiver Support

4th Angel
https://4thangel.ccf.org

Cancer 101
https://cancer101.org

Cancer Hope Network
https://cancerhopenetwork.org

Family Caregiver's Alliance
https://www.caregiver.org

Today's Caregiver
https://caregiver.com

Well Spouse
https://wellspouse.org

Children's Support

Alex's Lemonade Stand Foundation
www.alexslemonade.org

American Childhood Cancer Organization
www.acco.org

Andre Sobel River of Life Foundation
www.changingthepresent.org

Chase After a Cure
https://chaseafteracure.com

Children's Brain Tumor Foundation
https://cbtf.org

Children's Wish Foundation International
www.childrenswish.org

Clayton Dabney for Kids with Cancer
www.claytondabney.org

Cure Search for Children's Cancer
https://curesearch.org

Dream Factory
www.dreamfactoryinc.org

Emily Whitehead Foundation
https://emilywhiteheadfoundation.org

Hugs for Brady Foundation
www.hugsforbrady.com

Insure Kids Now
www.insurekidsnow.gov

Leaps of Love
https://www.leapsoflove.org

Lending Hearts
https://www.lendinghearts.org

Locks of Love
www.locksoflove.org

Make-A-Wish
www.wish.org

Making Headway
https://makingheadway.org

Mattie Miracle Cancer Foundation
www.mattiemiracle.com

The National Children's Cancer Society
www.thenccs.org

The National Pediatric Cancer Foundation
www.nationalpcf.org

Oracle Health Foundation
www.oraclefoundation.org

Palermo Foundation
https://www.palermo-foundation.org

Ronald McDonald House Charities
www.rmhc.org

Sofia's Hope
www.sofiashope.org

A Special Wish Foundation Inc
www.aspecialwishfoundation.org

St. Baldrick's Foundation
https://www.stbaldricks.org

Sunshine Foundation
www.sunshinefoundation.org

Teen Cancer America
https://teencanceramerica.org

The Taylor Matthews Foundation
https://taylormatthewsfoundation.org

Walk With Sally
https://walkwithsally.org

Clinical Trials

Clinicaltrials.gov by the National Institute of Health
www.clinicaltrials.gov

Coalition of Cancer Cooperative Groups, Inc.
www.cancertrialshelp.org

National Institutes of Health

www.nih.gov/health/clinicaltrials/index.htm

Trialjectory
https://www.trialjectory.com

Complementary & Alternative Medicine

Believe Big
www.believebig.org

Beyond Conventional Cancer Therapies
www.bcct.ngo

National Center for Complementary and Alternative
Medicine (NCCAM)
https://www.nccih.nih.gov

Connecting & Communicating

American Cancer Society
www.cancer.org

American Society of Clinical Oncology
www.cancer.net

CancerCare
www.cancercare.org

Cancer Fight Club
https://cancerfightclub.com

Cancer Hope Network
www.cancerhopenetwork.org

Cancer Support Community
www.cancersupportcommunity.org

Caring Bridge
www.caringbridge.org

Coping University
www.copinguniversity.com

I Had Cancer
www.ihadcancer.com

Imerman Angels (matches patients to a survivor)
www.imermanangels.org

Livestrong
www.livestrong.org

Lotsa Helping Hands
www.lotsahelpinghands.com

Man Up to Cancer
https://www.manuptocancer.com

MyLifeLine Cancer Foundation
www.mylifeline.org

National Cancer Institute
www.cancer.gov

Reach to Recovery
https://reach.cancer.org/
Download app on Apple App Store or Google Play

Drugmaker Financial Assistance

Amgen Safety Net Foundation
www.amgensafetynetfoundation.com

AstraZeneca
www.astrazeneca-us.com/medicines/Affordability

Bristol-Myers Squibb Access Support
www.BMSAccessSupport.com

Genentech
www.genentech-access.com/patient/biooncology.html

Janssen Ortho
www.janssenprescriptionassistance.com

Lilly
www.lillycares.com

Merck & Co
www.merckaccessprogram.com

Novartis Pharmaceuticals Corporation
www.patientassistancenow.com

Pfizer Inc.
www.pfizerrxpathways.com

RxAssist
www.rxassist.org

Emotional Support

Cancer Support Community
www.cancersupportcommunity.org

Employment Issues

Cancer and Careers
www.cancerandcareers.org

Cancer Legal Resource Center
www.thedrlc.org

End-of-Life

Hospice Education Institute
www.hospiceworld.org

Inspiration Hospice
https://inspirationhospice.com

National Hospice Foundation
www.nationalhospicefoundation.org

Exercise

2Unstoppable
www.2unstoppable.org

Expenses

The Assistance Fund
www.tafcares.org

Benefits.gov
www.benefits.gov

Cancer Financial Assistance Coalition
www.cancerfac.org

Cancer Information Service
www.cancer.gov

Family Reach
www.familyreach.org

Friends of Man
www.friendsofman.org

Good days
www.mygooddays.org

The Health Well Foundation
www.healthwellfoundation.org

Hill-Burton Program
www.hrsa.gov/get-health-care/affordable/hill-burton/facilities.html

Patient Access Network Foundation
www.panfoundation.org

Patient Advocate Foundation
www.patientadvocate.org
www.copays.org

RXAssistance Programs

www.rxassistanceprograms.com

Rx Outreach
www.rxoutreach.org

Social Security Administration
www.ssa.gov/applyfordisability

Zichron Shlome Refuah Fund
www.zsrf.org

Facing Homelessness

Catholic Charities USA
www.catholiccharitiesusa.org

Family Promise
www.familypromise.org

National Health Care for the Homeless Council
www.nhchc.org

Financial Assistance

American Cancer Society
www.cancer.org

Accessia Health
www.accessiahealth.org

BenefitsCheckup
www.benefitscheckup.org

Cancer *Care,* Inc.

www.cancercare.org/financial

Cancer Financial Assistance Coalition
www.cancerfac.org

Disability Rights Legal Center
www.thedrlc.org

Fund Finder
https://fundfinder.panfoundation.org

Give Forward
(Fundraising for your medical expenses)
www.giveforward.com

Good Days
www.mygooddays.org

HealthWell Foundation
www.healthwellfoundation.org

Hill-Burton Free Hospital Care
www.hrsa.gov/gethealthcare/affordable/hillburton

Lazarex Cancer Foundation
https://lazarex.org

Medicare Access for Patients RX
www.maprx.info

National Comprehensive Cancer Network
www.nccn.org

National Collegiate Cancer Foundation
https://collegiatecancer.org

NeedyMeds, Inc.
www.needymeds.org

NoWoodenNickels
www.nowoodennickels.org

Partnership for Prescription Assistance
www.pparx.org

Patient Access Network Foundation
www.panfoundation.org

Patient Advocate Foundation
www.patientadvocate.org

Rent Assistance
www.rentassistance.org

Supplemental Security Income (SSI)
www.ssa.gov/disabilityssi

U.S. Department of Veteran Affairs
www.va.gov

Financial Assistance Adolescents and Young Adults

Cameron Siemers Foundation for Hope
www.cameronsiemers.org

Cancer for College

www.cancerforcollege.org

Expect Miracles Foundation
www.expectmiraclesfoundation.org

Sofia's Hope
https://www.sofiashope.org/scholarships2

Financial Assistance by Disease

Blood

Be the Match
https://bethematch.org

Bone Marrow & Cancer Foundation
www.bonemarrow.org

Children's Leukemia Research Association
www.childrensleukemia.org

DKMS
https://www.dkms.org

Hairy Cell Leukemia
https://www.hairycellleukemia.org

Help Hope Live
www.helphopelive.org

Leukemia & Lymphoma Society
www.lls.org
Lymphoma Research Foundation

www.lymphoma.org/resources/supportservices/financ
ialsupport/

National CML Society
https://www.nationalcmlsociety.org

The Shannon Mosher Memorial Foundation
www.shannonmoshermemorial.com

Throwing Bones
https://throwing-bones.org

Brain Cancer

The Darren Daulton Foundation
www.darrendaultonfoundation.org

Friends4Michael Foundation
www.friends4michael.org

Glenn Garcelon Foundation
www.glenngarcelonfoundation.org

Matthew Larson Foundation for Pediatric Brain
Tumors
www.ironmatt.org/familyassistance

Mission4Maureen
www.mission4maureen.org

Owen Lea Foundation
www.owenleafoundation.org/assistance

Pediatric Brain Tumor Scholarship Foundation

www.curethekids.org/family-resources/scholarships

Thompson-Mason Brain Cancer Foundation
www.braincancerhelp.org

Breast

American Breast Cancer Foundation
www.abcf.org

The Donna Foundation
www.thedonnafoundation.org

Driving Miss Darby Foundation
www.drivingmissdarby.org/assistance

My Hope Chest
www.myhopechest.org

The Pink Daisy Project
www.pinkdaisyproject.com

The Pink Fund
https://pinkfund.org/

Rethink Breast Cancer
https://rethinkbreastcancer.com

Sisters Network Inc
www.sistersnetworkinc.org

United Breast Cancer Foundation
www.ubcf.org/programs/

Colorectal

Meredith's Miracles Colon Cancer Foundation
www.merediths-miracles.org

Fertility Preservation

Alliance for Fertility Preservation
https://www.allianceforfertilitypreservation.org

Livestrong Fertility
https://www.livestrong.org/what-we-do/program/fertility

The Oncofertility Consortium
https://oncofertility.msu.edu

Team Maggie for a Cure
www.teammaggieforacure.org/grants

Gastrointestinal Stromal Tumor

GIST Support International
www.gistsupport.org

Gynecological

Cancer Schmancer Movement
www.cancerschmancer.org

Foundation for Women's Cancer
https://www.foundationforwomenscancer.org/

HOPE in Oklahoma

https://hope.ouhsc.edu/

Society of Gynecologic Oncology
https://www.sgo.org/

Kidney

American Kidney Fund
www.kidneyfund.org

Liver

American Liver Foundation
www.liverfoundation.org

Pancreatic

National Pancreatic Cancer Foundation
www.npcf.us

Rare Cancers

National Organization for Rare Disorders
www.rarediseases.org/patient-assistance-programs

Sarcoma

Kylee's Dancing Angels
www.kyleesdancingangels.org

Sarcoma Alliance
www.sarcomaalliance.org/resources/financial-
assistance/

Strike Out for Sarcoma
www.dukehealth.org

Skin

Miles Against Melanoma
www.milesagainstmelanoma.com/family-assistance-
program

Stomach

Stomach Cancer Relief Network
www.scrnet.org

Financial Assistance for Older and Disabled Patients

BenefitsCheckUp
www.benefitscheckup.org

Medicare
www.medicare.gov

Medicare Rights Center
www.medicarerights.org

Financial Assistance for the Uninsured

Blink Health
www.blinkhealth.com

Medicaid
www.medicaid.gov
Partnership for Prescription Assistance
www.pparx.org

Veterans Benefits Administration
www.benefits.va.gov/benefits/

Government Aid

Administration for Children and Families HHS.gov
www.acf.hhs.gov

Hereditary

Bright Pink
www.brightpink.org

Facing Our Risk of Cancer Empowered, Inc (FORCE)
www.facingourrisk.org

Genetic Alliance, Inc
www.geneticalliance.org

Home Relief

CareCalendar
www.carecalendar.org

Cleaning for a Reason
www.cleaningforareason.org

Hotlines

American Cancer Society (ACS)
www.cancer.org

Bloch Cancer Hotline
www.blochcancer.org

Cancer *Care,* Inc.
www.cancercare.org

Image

Breast Friends Hat Project
https://breastfriends.org/request-a-hat/

EBeauty Community Inc.
www.ebeauty.com

Good Wishes
www.goodwishesscarves.org

Heavenly Hats Foundation
www.heavenlyhats.org

Knitted Knockers
www.knittedknockers.org

Lolly's Locks
www.lookgoodfeelbetter.org

Wigs & Wishes
www.wigsandwishes.org

Intimacy

American Association of Sexuality Educators,
Counselors and Therapists

www.aasect.org

Legal Support

Cancer Legal Resource Center
www.thedrlc.org/cancer

CancerLinc
www.cancerlinc.org

Know Cancer
www.knowcancer.com/cancer-lawyers

Law Help
www.lawhelp.org

Legal Aid Societies
www.lsc.gov

Patient Advocate Foundation
www.patientadvocate.org

Triage Cancer
https://triagecancer.org

LGBTQ Support

GLMA: Gay & Lesbian Medical Association
www.glma.org

National LGBT Cancer Network
www.cancer-network.org

Lymphedema

National Lymphedema Network
www.lymphnet.org

Medical Specialty Societies

American Association of Cancer Research
www.aacr.org

American College of Radiology
www.acr.org

American College of Surgeons
www.facs.org

American Society of Clinical Oncology (ASCO)
https://www.asco.org/

American Society of Hematology
www.hematology.org

American Society of Plastic Surgeons
www.plasticsurgery.org

American Society of Radiation Oncology
www.astro.org

National Society of Genetic Counselors
www.nsgc.org

Nonprofit Funding for Cancer Care and Living

The Assistance Fund
www.tafcares.org

Nutrition

American Institute for Cancer Research
https://www.aicr.org/

The Cancer Project
www.pcrm.org/health-topics/cancer

Oncology Massage Therapists

Society for Oncology Massage
www.s4om.org

Pain

American Chronic Pain Association
www.theacpa.org

PAPR Coalition
www.paprcoalition.com

Periodicals

Coping with Cancer Magazine
www.copingmag.com

Cure Magazine
www.curetoday.com

Patient Resource Cancer Guide
www.patientresource.com
aWomansHealth Magazine
https://awomanshealth.com/

Pregnancy and Fertility

Hope for Two. . .The Pregnant with Cancer Network
www.hopefortwo.org

Religious Support

Endurance with Jan and Dave Dravecky
https://www.endurance.org/

Inheritance of Hope
https://inheritanceofhope.org/

Sharsheret (Jewish)
www.sharsheret.org

Research

American Association for Cancer Research
www.aacr.org

Cancer Research Institute
www.cancerresearch.org

National Cancer Institute (NCI)
www.cancer.gov

Retreats/Camps
(Most of the retreats are free or charge low fees. Call to learn more.)

Base 2 Summit
https://cassiehinesshoescancer.org/base-2-summit

Betty J. Borry Breast Cancer Retreats

https://bjbbreastcancerretreats.org/

Camp Mak-A-Dream
www.campdream.org

Camp Good Days and Special Times
www.campgooddays.org

Casting for Recovery
https://castingforrecovery.org/

Commonweal Cancer Help Program
www.commonweal.org

Epic Experience
https://www.epicexperience.org/

First Descents
www.firstdescents.org

Healing Odyssey
www.healingodyssey.org

Hole in the Wall Gang Camp
www.holeinthewallgang.org

Kesem
https://www.kesem.org/

Kokolulu Farm and Cancer Retreat
www.cancer-retreat.org

Live by Living

www.livebyliving.org

Project Koru
www.projectkoru.org

Smith Farm Center: Cancer Help Program
www.smithfarm.com

Still Waters
https://www.stillwaterscancerretreat.org

Stowe Weekend of Hope
www.stowehope.org

True North Treks
https://www.truenorthtreks.org

Young Adult Cancer Canada
https://youngadultcancer.ca

Sleep

National Sleep Foundation
www.sleepfoundation.org

Survivorship

Livestrong Foundation
www.livestrong.org
National Coalition for Cancer Survivorship
www.canceradvocacy.org

Transportation — Affordable Accommodations

American Cancer Society Hope Lodge
https://www.cancer.org/support-programs-and-services/patient-lodging.html

Fisher House Foundation
https://fisherhouse.org

Joe's House
https://www.joeshouse.org

Hotel Keys for Hope
https://www.extendedstayamerica.com/acs-partnership

Healthcare Hospitality Network
https://www.hhnetwork.org/

Ronald McDonald House Charities
www.rmhc.org

Ryan House
www.ryanhouse.org

Transportation — Travel

Air Care Alliance
www.aircarealliance.org

Air Charity Network
www.aircharitynetwork.org

American Cancer Society's Road to Recovery
https://www.cancer.org/support-programs-and-services/road-to-recovery.html

Angel Flight
www.angelflight.com

Children's Flight of Hope
https://www.childrensflightofhope.org

Corporate Angel Network, Inc
www.corpangelnetwork.org

Lifeline Pilots
www.lifelinepilots.org

Mercy Medical Angels
www.mercymedical.org

Miracle Flights for Kids
www.miracleflights.org

Operation Liftoff
www.operationliftoff.org

PALS SkyHope
https://palservices.org

Uber Health
https://www.uberhealth.com/

Wigs, Hats, and Headgear

Breast Friends Hat Project
www.breastfriends.org

Heavenly Hats
https://heavenlyhats.org

Hope Scarves
www.hopescarves.org

Look Good. . . Feel Better
www.lookgoodfeelbetter.org

Wigs and Wishes by Maritino Cartier
www.wigsandwishes.org

Wigs for Kids
www.wigsforkids.org

<u>Young Adults</u>

ANCAN
https://ancan.org

Beads of Courage
https://beadsofcourage.org

Planet Cancer (Livestrong Foundation)
www.planetcancer.org

Dear Jack Foundation
https://www.dearjackfoundation.org

Elephants and Tea
https://elephantsandtea.com

Stupid Cancer
www.stupidcancer.org

Teenage Cancer Trust (UK)
www.teenagecancertrust.org

The Ruth Cheatham Foundation
https://www.ruthcheathamfoundation.org

The Cassie Hines Shoes Cancer Foundation
https://cassiehinesshoescancer.org

Ulman Foundation
https://ulmanfoundation.org

Young Adult Survivors United
https://www.yasurvivors.org

Disease Specific Resources

Bladder

American Bladder Cancer Society
https://bladdercancersupport.org/

Bladder Cancer Advocacy Network
www.bcan.org

Bladder Cancer WebCafe
www.blcwebcafe.org

Blood

Aplastic Anemia & MDS International Foundation

https://www.aamds.org

Be the Match
www.bethematch.org

Blood and Marrow Transplant Information Network
www.bmtinfonet.org

CLL Society
www.cllsociety.org

Cutaneous Lymphoma Foundation
www.clfoundation.org

DKSM
https://www.dkms.org

International Myeloma Foundation
https://www.myeloma.org/

International Waldenstrom's Macroglublinemia
Foundation
www.iwmf.com

The Leukemia & Lymphoma Society
www.lls.org

Lymphoma Research Foundation
https://lymphoma.org/

MPN Cancer Connection
https://mpncancerconnection.org

MPN Education Foundation
https://mpninfo.org

Multiple Myeloma Research Foundation
www.themmrf.org

Brain

American Brain Tumor Association
www.abta.org

Brain Tumour Foundation of Canada
https://www.braintumour.ca

Brain Tumor Network
www.braintumornetwork.org

Children's Brain Tumor Foundation
www.cbtf.org

EndBrainCancer Initiative
www.endbraincancer.org

Greg's Mission
www.gregsmission.org

International Brain Tumour Alliance
https://theibta.org

Musella Foundation for Brain Tumor Research &
Information
https://virtualtrials.org/
National Brain Tumor Society

www.braintumor.org

Pediatric Brain Tumor Foundation
www.akidsbraintumorcure.org

Tug McGraw Foundation
www.tugmcgraw.org

Breast

American Breast Cancer Foundation
https://www.abcf.org

Breastcancer.org
https://www.breastcancer.org/

Breast Cancer Trials
https://www.breastcancertrials.org/BCTIncludes/index
.html

Bright Pink
https://www.brightpink.org/

The Donna Foundation
https://thedonnafoundation.org/
https://breastcancermarathon.com/

EraseIBC
https://www.eraseibc.org
The IBC Network Foundation
www.theibcnetwork.org

Living Beyond Breast Cancer
https://www.lbbc.org/

Male Breast Cancer Coalition
www.malebreastcancercoalition.org

Metaplastic Breast Cancer
https://www.mpbcalliance.org

Metastatic Breast Cancer Alliance
https://www.mbcalliance.org

Metastatic Breast Cancer Network
http://mbcn.org/

MetAvivor
https://www.metavivor.org/

National Breast Cancer Foundation, Inc.
https://www.nationalbreastcancer.org/

Pink Chose Me
https://pinkchoseme.org/

Share Cancer Support
https://www.sharecancersupport.org

Sharsheret
https://sharsheret.org

Surviving Breast Cancer
https://www.survivingbreastcancer.org

Susan G. Komen
https://www.komen.org/

The Julie Fund
https://juliefund.org

Tigerlily Foundation
https://www.tigerlilyfoundation.org

Touch, The Black Breast Cancer Alliance
https://touchbbca.org

Triple Negative Breast Cancer Foundation
https://tnbcfoundation.org

Twisted Pink
https://www.twistedpink.org

Young Survival Coalition
https://youngsurvival.org/

Metastatic Breast

Metastatic Breast Cancer Network
http://mbcn.org/

Colorectal

AliveAndKickn
www.aliveandkickn.org

Colon Cancer Coalition
https://coloncancercoalition.org

Colon Cancer Foundation
https://coloncancerfoundation.org

Colon Club
https://www.colonclub.com/

Colorectal Cancer Alliance
https://www.ccalliance.org/

Fight Colorectal Cancer
https://fightcolorectalcancer.org/

Man Up to Cancer
https://www.manuptocancer.com

Raymond Foundation
https://www.theraymondfoundation.org/

Esophagus

Esophageal Cancer Awareness Association
https://www.ecaware.org/

Esophageal Cancer Education Foundation
https://fightec.org/

Gastrointestinal Stromal Tumor

GIST Support International
www.gistsupport.org

Gynecological

Bright Pink

https://www.brightpink.org

Clearity Foundation
https://www.clearityfoundation.org

Foundation for Women's Cancer
https://foundationforwomenscancer.org/

Gynecologic Cancer Foundation
http://www.thegcf.org/

National Cervical Cancer Coalition
https://www.nccc-online.org/

National Ovarian Cancer Coalition
https://ovarian.org/

Ovarian Cancer Research Alliance
https://ocrahope.org/

Share Cancer Support
https://www.sharecancersupport.org

Sharsheret
https://sharsheret.org

The Julie Fund
https://juliefund.org

Head and Neck

Head and Neck Cancer Alliance
https://headandneck.org/

The Oral Cancer Foundation
https://oralcancerfoundation.org/

Support for People with Oral & Head & Neck Cancer
https://spohnc.org/

<u>Kidney</u>

KCCure
https://kccure.org

Kidney Cancer Association
https://www.kidneycancer.org/

KidneyCAN
https://kidneycan.org

National Kidney Foundation
https://www.kidney.org/

<u>Liver</u>

Blue Faery
www.bluefaery.org

American Liver Foundation
https://liverfoundation.org/

Cholangiocarcinoma Foundation
https://cholangiocarcinoma.org/

Fibrolamellar Cancer Foundation
https://fibrofoundation.org/
Global Liver Institute

https://globalliver.org/

Yes
http://www.beatlivertumors.org/

Lung

ALK Positive
https://www.alkpositive.org

American Lung Association
https://www.lung.org/lung-force

Bonnie J. Addario Lung Cancer Foundation
www.lungcancerfoundation.org

Free to Breathe
https://www.lungcancerresearchfoundation.org/get-involved/free-to-breathe/

GO2 For Lung Cancer
https://go2.org

KRAS Kickers
https://www.kraskickers.org

LiveLung
https://livelung.org/

Lung Cancer Alliance
https://go2.org/

Lung Cancer Research Foundation

https://www.lungcancerresearchfoundation.org

LUNGevity Foundation
https://www.lungevity.org/

Met Crusaders
https://metcrusaders.org/

The Chris Draft Family Foundation
http://www.chrisdraftfamilyfoundation.org

Upstage Lung Cancer
https://upstagelungcancer.org

Lynch Syndrome

AliveAndKickn
www.aliveandkickn.org

Neuroendocrine

Neuroendocrine Cancer Awareness Network
https://www.netcancerawareness.org/

Neuroendocrine Tumor Research Foundation
https://netrf.org/

The Healing Net Foundation
https://www.thehealingnet.org/

Oral

SPOHNC: Support for People with Oral,
https://spohnc.org/

Pancreas

Let's Win Pancreatic Cancer
https://letswinpc.org/

Lustgarten Foundation
https://lustgarten.org

Pancreatic Cancer Action Network
https://pancan.org/

National Pancreas Foundation
https://pancreasfoundation.org/

National Pancreatic Cancer Foundation
https://www.npcf.us/

Prostate

Fans for the Cure
https://fansforthecure.org

National Alliance of State Prostate Cancer Coalitions
https://naspcc.org

Prostate Cancer Foundation
https://www.pcf.org/
Prostate Cancer Research Institute
www.pcri.org

Prostate Conditions Education Council
https://www.prostateconditions.org
USTOO Prostate International Education and Support

https://zerocancer.org/

Zero
https://zerocancer.org

Sarcoma

National Leiomyosarcoma Foundation
https://nlmsf.org/

Sarcoma Alliance
https://sarcomaalliance.org/

Sarcoma Foundation of America
https://www.curesarcoma.org/

Skin

A Cure in Sight
https://acureinsight.org

Aim at Melanoma
https://www.aimatmelanoma.org/

Melanoma Research Foundation
https://melanoma.org/

Skin Cancer Education & Research Foundation
https://skincancerinfo.org

Skin Cancer Foundation
www.skincancer.org

Stomach/Gastric

Debbie's Dream Foundation: Curing Stomach Cancer
https://debbiesdream.org/

GI Cancer Alliance
https://www.gicancersalliance.org

Hope for Stomach Cancer
https://stocan.org/

No Stomach for Cancer
https://nostomachforcancer.org/

Testicular

Testicular Cancer Awareness Foundation
www.testicularcancerawarenessfoundation.org

Testicular Cancer Foundation
https://www.testicularcancer.org

Thyroid

ThyCa: Thyroid Cancer Survivor's
https://www.thyca.org/

ThyTabono
https://thytabono.org

ACKNOWLEDGMENTS

This is the part of the book where the author thanks all the people who tirelessly proofread the manuscript, the friends who loaned their beach house for the author to escape and write, the mentor who they emailed "What do I do??" or "What do you recommend?" on a continuous basis, and the many friends who provided invaluable feedback throughout the process – as if they had any damn choice in the matter. There's also usually some kind of note to the spousal unit, who remained patient and loving during the entire time the book was being written and with whom the author is probably still arguing about the time and money spent to make it all happen, and the kids who gave their opinion and feedback but the author didn't listen and did it their own way anyways.

But none of this is of any importance, because nobody ever reads this pointless page anyways.